Awake in the World

Awake in the World

TEACHINGS FROM YOGA & BUDDHISM
FOR LIVING AN ENGAGED LIFE

MICHAEL STONE

Shambhala

BOSTON & LONDON

2011

Shambhala Publications, Inc.
Horticultural Hall
300 Massachusetts Avenue
Boston, Massachusetts 02115
www.shambhala.com

9 8 7 6 5 4 3 2 1

First Edition
Printed in the United States of America

♾This edition is printed on acid-free paper that meets the
American National Standards Institute z39.48 Standard.
♻This book was printed on 30% postconsumer recycled paper.
For more information please visit www.shambhala.com.

Distributed in the United States by Random House, Inc.,
and in Canada by Random House of Canada Ltd

Designed by Katrina Noble

Library of Congress Cataloging-in-Publication Data
Stone, Michael (Michael Jason), 1974–
Awake in the World: Teachings from Yoga and Buddhism for
Living an Engaged Life / Michael Stone.—First Edition.
p. cm.
ISBN 978-1-59030-814-1 (pbk.)
1. Yoga. 2. Religious life—Buddhism. I. Title.
B132.Y6S7635 2011
181′.45—dc22

To Arlyn and the Centre of Gravity Sangha

May your eye go to the sun, your life's breath to the wind.
Go to the sky or earth, as is your nature; or go to the waters
   if that is your fate.
Take root in the plants with all your limbs.

—RG Veda

CONTENTS

Contents

SANSKRIT PRONUNCIATION

I'VE OFFERED diacritical marks throughout the text to help you familiarize yourself with common terms in the Yoga tradition. The following is a simple guide to pronouncing these Sanskrit terms.

There are five Sanskrit diacritic markings in the text:
A line above the letter (ā)
A dot above the letter (ṅ)
A dot below the letter (ḍ)
A tilde above the letter (ñ)
An acute accent above the letter (ś)

VOWELS

a (short) is like the *a* in *sofa,* as in the word *manas* (mind).
ā (long) is like the *a* in *psalm,* as in *āsana* (posture).
au is like the *ou* in *out,* as in *Gautama Buddha.*
i (short) is like the *i* in *knit,* as in *cit* (consciousness).
ī (long) is like the *ee* in *meet,* as in *jīva* (soul).
u (short) is like the *u* in *put,* as in *guṇa* (quality or attribute).
ū (long) is like the *u* in *rule,* as in *rūpa* (form).

CONSONANTS

c is like the *ch* in *church* and never pronounced like *k* in *car* or *s* in *sent.* An example of this is *cakra* or *cit.*

ñ is palatal and nasal, like the *ny* in *canyon* or the *ni* in *onion*, and this is how a name such as *Patañjali* is pronounced.

ṛ is pronounced like the *ri* in *rivet*, and is usually found in *Kṛṣṇa*.

ṅ or *ṁ* is like the *n* in *uncle*, as found in the words *saṅgha* or *saṁskāra*.

ṣ and *ś* are pronounced as *sh*, though the tongue position of *ś* is palatal as in the word *shock*, and the tongue position of *ṣ* has the tip of the tongue at the roof of the mouth, as found in the English *shun* and the romanized Sanskrit word *ṣunyata*.

Although Sanskrit words are not pluralized by adding an *s* the way English words are, we've used the *s* in such terms as *āsanas*, in order to ease readability in English.

PREFACE

Between 2004 and 2010, almost all of the talks I gave, from Copenhagen to Costa Rica to Cape Cod to California, were recorded in one form or another. Every once in a while, someone would send me something he or she had recorded or notated. In the meantime, friends and strangers have transcribed this collection of talks, which includes lectures in academic settings, formal talks on retreat, and weekly community meetings with Centre of Gravity Sangha in Toronto. I hope these words are encouraging and provoking. The Yoga tradition is primarily oral, and I hope that even though many of these talks were offered in formal settings, the spirit of community debate, shared practice, and ongoing inquiry comes vividly through these pages.

Yoga comes alive in *this* culture at *this* time only when we integrate committed practice with the kind of community-based inquiry that puts practice to work both individually and collectively. These teachings come from a nonhierarchal approach to teaching that replaces the teacher/expert at the front of the room and the student/ seeker as audience with a democratic "open-source" style of learning where lectures give way to open debate and group practice.

There is nothing holy or religious about Yoga theory or practice. These teachings are most alive in the gardens, alleys, and ravines where those who may not even know they are yogis are challenging the status quo both internally and externally. This is not a practice that thrives in temples or commercial studios. This is a path for those seeking freedom from the psychological and cultural entanglements of mind and body. I hope these talks will encourage you to bring your practice to a deeper level by placing it at the center of your life rather than the outskirts of your lifestyle. We are living in times of personal, social, ecological, and economic imbalance. These talks are designed to steer your Yoga practice in a direction that integrates the formal path (on the cushion, on the mat, in the meditation hall) with the everyday activities of one's day-to-day life (cooking, cleaning, communicating) in such a way that any practice dualities dissolve. In the same way that all freshwater rivers reach toward the saline oceans, your life and your Yoga practice are seamless continuities of one another. Though Yoga practices such as postures and sitting and breathing techniques sometimes feel like activities separated from daily life, this book is designed to clarify such distinctions so that your every action becomes an expression of Yoga. May this collection be of benefit to you personally as well as to the great watersheds, architecture, cities, biota, and forests that nourish us and desperately need our creative attention.

Om Shanti

PART ONE

Practicing Inward and Outward

1

This Is It

The Here and Now of Everyday Living

I came to realize clearly that mind is nothing other than
mountains and rivers and the great wide earth, the sun
and the moon and the stars.
—DOGEN, *Shobogenzo*

IT IS NOT NECESSARY for you to try too hard in this practice.
All that is necessary is for your mind and body to be present like
the moving grasses, the petals of a tulip, the currents and subcurrents
of endless rivers. Take your concepts of the body composed of all the
elements, your concept of the mind composed by the past, your self-
image, and cast them off, beyond the world of form. Until we drop
our concepts and efforts in this practice, it's difficult to value the fact
that "this is it." There is nothing special to become or achieve.

The Buddha reminds us that we need to move beyond our fantasies of permanence and eternal salvation in some future existence
and instead open to the always-changing cascade of life that we call
reality. The body as it manifests in the here and now—with pupils
dilating, stomach acids churning, and veins pulsing—and the breath
as it arises and passes away along the inner walls of the septum teach

us something about the provisional ground of reality. We are not concerned, in Yoga, with some ultimate reality. We are concerned with the way things happen in each and every moment. Within this awareness we can open to a vivid and still calm at the root of all experience. In the absence of turmoil, greed, and self-reference, we experience deep *samādhi*—the embodied vividness of nonseparation. *Samādhi* is not a permanent achievement or final state in which you rest outside the temporal and unreliable flow of conditioned life. *Samādhi* is a glimpse, even if sustained over a period of time, of the ground in which one recognizes that one is free to be in this world without being gripped by exaggeration, craving, or rejection. It is the carving out of a path from the provisional ground of our body, gender, family, and overall circumstances. This is freedom from being pushed and pulled by habitual drives. It is certainly not turning away from the world. Even the ground is groundless. The ground we stand on is always moving, and new actions are always required. Every time we arrive at a new viewpoint, the conditions change, and we must once again tune in to what is under our feet. The possibility opens, in this groundless ground, to move through the world with love and lucidity. Love becomes both the perceptive quality of awareness and the motivating force behind our actions. But loving action is possible only in the absence of a contracted viewpoint (*avidyā*). Again, we are not trying to find an ultimate view; we are practicing techniques that help us relinquish our contraction around views so that we can tune in to how life happens.

Pre-Buddhist and pre-Patañjali Yoga are both concerned with looking beyond the here and now for salvation, whether in the form of the *ātman* (soul), *jīva* (eternal self), or Brahman (origin of the manifest). This kind of approach to liberation leads one into the beyond, the future, and shuts down the value of the immediate here and now. It's not that the language of "soul" or "self" is problematic in and of itself; the difficulty arises when we are looking outside of ourselves for salvation or liberation.

Yogic awareness is the literal yoking of our attention (*citta*) to what is actually going on in the ordinary vicissitudes of each and every moment.

In your own practice, I encourage you not to lead with your belief system but to investigate physical reality prior to metaphysical speculation.

There is some desire in every one of us—of every race and color and background—to draw lines in the sand of our lives and defend these boundaries as if these conditioned beliefs were somehow eternally true. *Avidya* (not seeing things as they are) draws us into a kind of defensive situation where we are trying to match what's happening with what we want to happen. So much of what I call my life is only happening as snapshots in my imagination. The body and the world are movements I cannot catch up with. Life, and this very body and self, are not fixed in this way. We are rhizomatic, we are split atoms spreading out from a core, we are fluid creatures in every sense. Seeing life and death in this body and breath and in everything we do allows us to let go of clinging. Every attempt by the brain and muscles to capture what moves through our senses is always inadequate. The world is too large, and in constant flux, for us to draw conclusions. The best we can do is to enter life in such a way that we see that our ideas are only fading snapshots we string together, as brief as a breath.

Sometimes I am a father hanging out at the skateboard park with my son, picking him up when he falls and helping him learn new tricks. Hours later, when he is away from me and I wander through the same park with friends, or sit at my favorite bustling coffee shop to read while he's at school, I don't experience myself as a father, I move through the world in an entirely different way. Identity is a spectrum, and in varying conditions, who and what I am shifts. Even the body is made of elements found in the natural world that we can hardly call "ours." Whether I think in terms of identity, ecology, or gender, "I" am an endless possibility, a million characters coming to being. Truth is always shifting. It's not until we see through our preoccupation with having a viewpoint that we can genuinely listen to a given situation and take appropriate loving action. Shifting life always swallows and absorbs every viewpoint eventually. This is what makes practice so important. Without training the mind to see through its own preoccupations, it becomes hard to tune in to what each situation requires from us. Can we stop and put our viewpoint aside in order to really bear witness to what's happening in and around us? This dynamic of pausing and opening to a wider view works the same internally as it does socially and politically.

Training begins with learning how to open the channels of the body through the Yoga postures, and then following through with sitting meditation, where the energy from the posture practice can settle the nerves and mind. Unlike when we practice the Yoga postures, in sitting meditation we simply open to what is moving through the body without moving into it or away from it. We open to experience from a place of stillness.

If there is no fixed enlightenment, we must keep asking: What is this now? It's the "now" that is important. It's the "what" that is secondary. You don't need to answer the question. The "what" orients us toward the now. But the now is not separate from you. The now is endless time—you become time when you become yourself. There is no "outside," no "me" in time or "you" outside time; we are always time as we are always ourselves. When we are fully in a moment, time dissolves into a more rhythmic sequence: the body ages, the sun moves across the sky, we become hungry and prepare a meal. There is a relationship between being fully in our lives and losing track of time in the narrow sense. When we are overburdened with stress, time becomes a condition we struggle with. And yet we all know the feeling of being free in time, not caught up in the worry of getting through an hour or a day.

A red finch flies by the window. Then another follows her call. The finch isn't thinking about being a finch or flying through time. The finch is a function of the natural world, and the sound of a bird shares the same bandwidth as your voice. What does it mean to be a sentient being? What is it to be you in the same way the finch is herself?

Samādhi means integrity that is more than being true to yourself. It is exactly what the finch is doing but applied in the human realm. We are not finches. It is effectively integrating one's self in one's social, economic, cultural, familial, and ecological contexts. At this level, integrity is the ground in which self and culture mutually arise for maximum benefit. For love. For the flourishing of all beings.

To capture this in words, I would need run-on sentences so long that they would begin in the rivers and end in the skies. I wish language could do that. Sometimes I hear my son repeating words and phrases I've said to him and catch my own forms of expression moving through his small mind and body.

Sometimes I try to speak about practice in ways that are so simple that all I want to say is: Pay attention to inhaling and exhaling without adding any theory or thought And then at other times, I want to participate in the rigorous discourse of academia, the development of psychological theory, and the highbrow conversations going on within intellectual communities. This seems like a paradox, and I'm learning that it comes through in my speech, my writing, and the ways I think about what I do when I am alone reflecting on the different hats I wear in one week. I have never wanted to be a Yoga teacher limited to teaching headstands or a clinician always working behind closed doors. I try to integrate the simplicity and stillness earned through attention to breathing or tracing circling birds and light snow, and then I jump into dialogue with anticapitalist activists or theologians about the ways Yoga philosophy can contribute to a better world. I struggle trying to integrate these sides of myself and the many practices that Yoga can offer me in this multifaceted world.

USING THE TOOLS OF PRACTICE

The direction of this practice points back to each one of us. This body and heart are not only what we study but also what we use as tools for living an engaged life. This body and heart can be tools for peacemaking. But they are only valuable tools when they have vitality and energy. We study ourselves so that we can move beyond the self. What you want to learn about is you. When you study this "you" closely, you start to disappear. Even if you find a terrible person inside you, if you look at it closely, it doesn't stand up. Nothing really does. At bottom, we cannot be reduced to one thing. Even spikes of craving only last for a few minutes at a time. Because our cravings and addictions can be so exhausting, it's important that we learn from them and transform these old habits so we can become useful tools for social change. We practice both for ourselves and for our culture at large.

So then how do we understand ourselves? We embody the practice in order to go out into the world. The most important thing I've felt in my years of practice is that we are not alone. Liberation is not dependent on the form of practice but on recognizing interdependence. When the Buddha taught that the self is simply an interdependent matrix, he set the stage for a socially engaged dharma practice. If what we are in every sense is everything within and around us, our every action makes a difference. When we see this body as a tool for social benefit, we begin to take care of it as we take care of our Earth. And we take care of the earth as we take care of our body.

We know we are all connected, but we forget. We know mind and body are one, but we wake every morning with amnesia. This is why we practice. We use this practice as a tool to effect change internally and externally in this very imbalanced world. The eighth-century Chinese Zen master Baizhang Huaihai clarifies this point in a dialogue with his dharma friend Yunyan, who went on to be an ancestor of the Soto Zen school:

> Yunyan asked, "Every day we have hard work. For whom do we do it?"
> Baizhang said, "There is someone who requires it."
> Yunyan said, "Why not let that person do it?"
> Baizhang said, "He has no tools."[1]

We need tools: to learn to sit still, to turn self-centeredness into altruistic action, to take care of ourselves and our communities. Through expressing Yoga in everything we do, we instill in others the tools necessary for their own inner and outer work. Our practice becomes a social tool for others.

How do we live a balanced life in an unbalanced time? How does our practice help us to maintain the sensory equanimity we need to participate effectively in our families and communities? The key to this life of practice is the heart that propels this process. The value of this work lies in our own heart, the heart of the world.

Guelph, Ontario, 2008

2

Reading the Sky
for Weather Signs

When the blackbird flew out of sight,
It marked the edge
Of one of many circles.
—WALLACE STEVENS, "THIRTEEN WAYS OF
LOOKING AT A BLACKBIRD"

I WAS WALKING through Union Square Farmers Market this morning, amazed at the number of birds flying overhead. The farmers were sipping on warm apple cider, and I stopped to speak to them about the market and comment on the birds. Coming out of the subway, I didn't even notice the birds until I saw two men sitting in the back of their truck watching the circling birds as they creased the sky overhead. When the whole body is listening and speaking, we forget about ourselves. When I was listening to the two men talk about the way the birds don't show until ten o'clock in the morning, I caught the clock in the distance and realized if I didn't get going I'd be late for the workshop. Losing track of time, forgetting about ourselves, and paying attention to what is near in each moment conspire to open us to what is. And sometimes we might be surprised at what shows up. The birds circle overhead, the winter gives way to spring, and New York City is waking up at dawn.

I went early to the farmers' market because I didn't sleep well last night. Perhaps it was because of a long travel day yesterday, but more honestly, it's hard to visit farmers' markets without my son. Before his mother and I separated, we'd wake early every Saturday and go to the farmers market in downtown Toronto and wander around for hours. We'd always lose track of time while going from stall to stall trying new cheeses and then always end with some strange invention for a drink. Last week my son asked the person at the juicer to make him something with beet, celery, and enough ginger to make the drink burst into flames. Today I ordered plain, hot cider. Talking with the farmers, my mood changed and I forgot about how I was feeling about my son, until now.

A few hours later and here I am with you, to be together for a few hours as a collaborative learning community. We can learn just as much from one another as we can from birds and apples and farmers at Union Square. This morning I learned about the way my mood shifts when I tune in to what's actually happening in my body and in my surroundings. And what are the birds doing up there? When one red-winged blackbird flew overhead, it looked straight at me and then up to the sky again, as if it were reading the sky for weather patterns and pointing out to me the good news.

The paradox is that even though we can enter life so thoroughly that we forget our habits and even ourselves for a while, we still operate in the realm of language and thought. We cannot live in some idealized "oneness" all the time, the mind simply doesn't work that way. Although we can experience moments of deep clarity and intimacy, we always return to the world of body, speech, and mind. We never get beyond form. We can never escape our bodies. The absolute self of interdependence and diverse life and the relative self of habit and thinking both share an equal place in a mature spiritual practice. Although we are part of every corner of the universe, we are also idiosyncratic, and uniquely so.

Yoga is the expression of intimacy in every one of our actions in three spheres: body, speech, and mind. Intimacy does not simply refer to sex. I translate the word *yoga* as "intimacy" to connote the fact that everything is inherently contingent on everything else, from the basic molecules and strings that hold the world together all the way to the familial bonds that give rise to families and character. When we see that interconnectedness runs through each and every thing that we encounter, we begin to see that entering our lives fully is the deepest kind of intimacy we can ever encounter. In fact, in order to heal, we need to find an intimate connection to whatever it is that ails us. To be intimate with pain, sadness, or even loneliness is to enter that state of mind fully. This doesn't mean becoming completely absorbed, obsessed, or wallowing. It means riding the lively wave of anxiety or joy until it disperses and becomes something else. So intimacy is not just pleasure or sex. Intimacy in the context of the dharma means being one with what is in our lives in this very moment.

If our practice is not activated in and through body, language, and thought, it's a fragmented practice that leaves out the essentials of our daily experience as humans. Even when I say these words, they are completed in your experience and then activated in your life. The way I speak, the way you listen, and the way we act all form an interconnected universe. This interconnected web of perception and action, mind and body, speech and listening, comes together and comes apart in each moment of flow that we call life.

Meditation, Yoga postures, breathing practices, and contemplation are too often thought to be the core of practice. If we consider these pursuits as solitary and private, we forget about the other side of being human: creative expression. We do not live in an ethical vacuum. Therefore, it's important that we practice Yoga in a way that lends itself both to the internal forms of practice and to the expression of Yoga in everything we do.

In some ways, the technical aspects of Yoga practice—sitting meditation, chanting, breathing sequences, Yoga posture refinement— are all solitary pursuits that we engage in on the outskirts of culture. Sometimes we imagine a monk in his cave far away from a movie theater or village square. I have never met a monk, priest, or teacher who is not fully immersed in his or her society. Cultural products such as arts and literature give meaning to our lives, and the old texts and meditation manuals are also cultural creations. Every religion comes through a society in a given time. Even religions are created and refined by humans. The yogi does not so much drop out of culture as drop deeply into a culture. By seeing through the individual and institutional patterns of greed, hatred, and confusion, the yogi becomes a tool for social change. She's learned to work with her capacity for anger and reactivity and in so doing has something very real to offer others.

Cultural forces impact our mind and body. The way we work with our own habits and potentials in turn serves our culture. Internal practices always flow back out into the world. And the outer world of film and music and pollution and celebration always flows through us in whatever we do. There is no way to separate individual and collective, internal or external.

There are methods that can help us move back and forth between the seemingly internal dimension of practice and the everyday demands of our world, especially the world of the householder. There can be no activity that is separable from the movement of the individual. Even when we bathe we are washing a small corner of the universe. When we work with our tendencies toward anger or competitiveness, greed or confusion, we are directly serving everything within and around us.

When I am upset, sometimes I ask myself: Why are you angry? Why are you afraid? And then I can listen until fear or anger presents its reasons. But usually I am impatient. I feel angry and want to blame someone or yell or tell someone what I think about him or her. This is exactly where practice comes in.

Our practice teaches us how to open to anger or any other strong feelings and not take immediate action. We learn to wait and see. And in this waiting we become deeply engaged with what is showing up. I can't seal myself off and hope against hope for the end of anger. Anger has a purpose. But I have a responsibility to work with that anger, because as a practitioner of this practice called intimacy, I vow to remember that I do not live in an ethical vacuum. And though anger makes me feel like the center of the universe, I am not.

THE BREATH AS A TOOL

Just as we read the sky for signs of weather and read books for helpful insights, the yogi begins in the body, combing through the knots and flows of the body as a way to ground the movements of mind and breath. To give attention to the birds, I also have to be fully in my body. Beginning with the breath, we drop down into the pelvis, flow as we exhale, and then become aware up across the collarbones as we inhale and the roof of the mouth domes up. The collarbones lift and spread horizontally, like the lintel of the throat, and the hollow mouth quiets any clamoring in the nerves. The complementary opposites of inhaling and exhaling turn the mind away from the magnetic pull of overthinking and overimagining. Returning to the arc of the full inhalation and exhalation, the mind comes back to neutrality, back to present experience.

Like returning to the same flowerbed in your backyard, season after season, following the breath is a return to a familiar though always changing Earth. Of course, the ground changes, yet there are enough features for us to recognize something secure. When we breathe down to the end of every exhalation, sensation appears in the pelvic floor, and then a natural pause occurs before the inhalation shows up. The pause goes by many names: *bāhya kumbhaka, apāna, mūla bandha, mūla dhāra cakra.* The pause is the empty space at the end of the breath. And it seems as though thoughts appear with inhalation and fade away during the exhalation. When we're attentive to the exhalation, thoughts disappear like chalk dust, like wind.

The end of the exhalation is a good place to be silent. Paradoxically, it's both our secure base and it's always going away. The roof of the mouth hollows at the end of the exhaling pattern and the breath itself engenders or gives rise to tone at the center of the pelvic diaphragm. This tone is a sensation of spreading at the corners of the pelvic floor and a natural drawing up above the perineum. It's quiet and easy to miss. The mind settles. This quiet space is a hundred thousand years of evolution at a standstill. It's the gap between thoughts, between time and space, between one "thing" and another. It's also the place of healing. When our attention (*citta*) bonds with the feeling of the breath (*prāṇa*) in the pelvic floor (*mūla bandha*), it's not possible to feel this and remain caught up in stories and distractions. The feeling at the end of an exhalation is a tool for concentration. What we enter at the end of an exhalation is a focused place of letting go. If there is sadness or agitation, anxiety or distraction, the end of an exhalation can be a very physical way of grounding our attention even in those turbulent states.

LETTING GO

The end of an exhale is a profound letting go. In that space of release we begin to see that everything we thought of as solid or permanent passes away and becomes something else. All of these words and theories and forms are empty. So are you. A text is not a static thing, and neither are these sentences and neither are you. Each of you will enact, represent, and express the Yoga teachings in your own unique way. In fact, all teachings are only viable if they can be lived. When we make the body, the Yoga postures, or even our self-image a fixed "thing" in time and space, we end up limiting the potential of these forms. Everything gets derailed. Nothing is definitive or fixed: not your identity, sexuality, movements, or thoughts. When you look at a wave and focus on a molecule or imagine you can distinguish a liter of water one hundred feet from the shore, it's fascinating to realize that that particular liter of water does not come in and crash on the shore. That liter of water just goes up and down. The waves are a sequential sharing of energy, not a static pattern moving forward toward the shore. Likewise, your habits and thoughts are not static. You are not a depressed person or a sad person. You are not schizophrenic or angry. All of our moods and identities are flowing waves that appear and dissolve in varied conditions. There is not a fixed "thing" continuing through these waves.

A wave is not wondering about the future. A wave is just receiving and flowing with its conditions. Unity or Yoga is not a metaphysical principle but attunement to the flow of life through us, as us. The body is flowing. Thoughts and feelings are also moving. Nothing is definitive. Nothing. In the *āsana* practice we are releasing into the breath until we become one with breathing, and the postures float along on the currents of breath. The postures are strung on the breath so that they are not completely willed but also not passive. In this way the Yoga practice involves your whole life, translating and retranslating the breath, mind, intention, and thought patterns. Waves flow into more waves, but a wave is never a static entity. Language is also a flow taking place through the body. Sentences are nodes and tissues and symbols of past experiences coming alive now. We are all inheritors of previous cultural achievements, and language is one of them. So in the same way we wake up the body through Yoga *āsana,* the breath through *prāṇāyāma,* the mind through quiet sitting and also through study, we need relationships with others to help activate the intelligence of speech and listening. The way the farmers in the pickup truck studied the birds brought me out of my mood and into their flow of attention. We can all have far better listening skills. We can also improve our ways of speaking so we are not repeating cultural or even institutionalized forms of greed, hierarchy, and confusion.

In the same way that the job of a good writer is to get the reader into the story by writing scenes and characters that the reader can interpret on his or her own, the job of the Yoga teacher is to step aside and help the student establish an appropriate and autonomous practice that changes over time. I encourage students to practice in both a solitary and social way, alternating between time alone with their Yoga mat and cushion and also time in their community serving others and practicing with others. Community and solitude support one another. When we can be at ease in our own hearts and bodies, it's easier to meet others. You don't even have to decide whether you are a social or a solitary person. We are all both. The point here is that if we are going to erase the artificial divide between spiritual practice and everything else, we have to live in a way that is undivided.

If we listen to life—and by *life* I am referring to ourselves, our intimates, as well as birds and rivers and traffic—we interrupt the habit-forming and habit-reinforcing tendency to create opposites: me and you, body and mind, speech and listening. A good conversation has a flow between listening and talking. Movement in the body has the flow between steadiness and ease. The breath is both a current of movement and the always-present anchor that roots us in the body in the present moment.

These teachings and practices that we call "Yoga" are merely instruments to help us return to the moment-to-moment unfoldings of rhizomatic life, which is life that leaves nothing out. Under carefully preserved tea leaves that traditional texts were encoded upon in libraries in Calcutta, within the complex dynamics of a modern household, within the delicate maneuvers of sexual relations, and within the struggles of our jobs, we can find a place where we feel connected. These teachings are about such a connection and the way the teachings form a path out of the moods, changes, and overall conditions of our lives.

When I walked to Union Square this morning, I really didn't notice how much those two farmers pulled me out of myself and into the larger world I inhabit. Within minutes I went from a contracted state of sadness and sentimentality to a freer state in which that sadness could inhabit the same sky as the birds.

The continuous fabric of the mind, the firing patterns of billions of neurons, the irregular and natural movements of the respiratory diaphragm, drinking cider, losing what we hold dear, sending e-mails to friends, all flow seamlessly into one unique life. This is our life. Let's not miss it.

New York City, March 2009

3

The Realization of Intimacy

When one does not cling to actions or to the sense-
objects and has renounced all compulsive intention
and expectation, then one is said to have awakened
to Yoga.
—BHAGAVAD-GĪTĀ VI.418

W E FIND A PATH by carving it out of the conditions of our
lives. Though we hope that religious practices and spiritual
teachings will draw us out of sorrow and into an eternally steady and
calm state, attention to the body anchors us in the actuality of present experience whether painful, lonely, sad, or joyful. Over time,
these teachings and practices bring about a less reactive and more
creative way of being in the world, though they cannot remove the
inevitable pain and difficulty that comes with being an engaged
human citizen. There is a wonderful story about Jñāndev and
Nāmdev, two pilgrims walking together and learning from each
other. As they share the road together, Jñāndev becomes inspired by
Nāmdev's simple renunciate life and begins questioning his own
path of knowledge and practice. He implores Nāmdev:

Nāmā, tell me how your Self became undifferentiated with the
divine, who is the embodiment of love. Pleasure and devotion

are unbreakably united in you. What are the details of your method? How do you practice it? Tell me. What rites do you observe? How do you maintain your intellectual activities? What is your way of stilling the mind through meditation? Give me some kind of answer to these questions. How does one hear about your way? How does one think about it? How do you become firm in your practice through concentrated effort? Who is the one that worships? Who is the one that teaches? Show me someone who takes up this occupation. I am giddy and impatient! I should get started fasting and practicing your method today! Tell me your experiences.[1]

Because Nāmdev does not feel he has the authority to speak, he remains silent and continues to walk his path for a while. Nāmdev's silence reminds us that our questions about practice and how to really enter our lives cannot be answered by an external authority. Although we may be pointed in a helpful direction by those around us, especially great teachers and guides and community, it's the intensity of our questioning and bewilderment that fuels our motivation to practice. I think of how many times I've gone to mentors, friends, or teachers with vexing questions like whether I should stay in or leave a challenging relationship. Some of the most powerful insights have come to me when the people with whom I am sharing are able to be quiet and simply hold a space for what I am feeling. They hold silence for places in me that at the time I could not hold quietly.

What are your questions? What motivates your practice? What is the path of Yoga?

Yoga provides a direct and precise recognition of the play of the mind and the way thought and self-clinging perpetuate feelings of anxiety and alienation in a world that is fundamentally connected. When I was studying psychoanalytic thought at the University of Toronto, I was caught between whether I should become an academic or leave school altogether. I imagined entering a monastic path where I could study and practice day in and day out. Every day I struggled back and forth between the academic path that could possibly offer me a route to writing and eventually a job, or the quiet life of wearing robes, meditating, and ringing bells. I felt that I *had* to decide what I was and what I would become. It was hard to hold a place where I was a more fluid person, not exactly an academic and not quite a monastic. Then I came across this passage by philosopher William James that I kept pinned above my desk for the following year.

> Now can we tell more precisely in what the feeling of the central active self consists? . . . First of all, I am aware of a constant play of furtherances and hindrances in my thinking. . . . Among the matters I think of, some range themselves on the side of the thought's interests [passions], whilst others play an unfriendly part thereto [aggression]. The mutual inconsistencies and agreements, reinforcement and obstructions . . . produce . . . incessant reactions of my spontaneity upon them, welcoming or opposing, appropriating or disowning, striving with or against, saying yes or no. This palpitating inward life is, in me, that central nucleus [of the self].[2]

Though I certainly found moments of quietude in my meditation practices at the time, I was relieved to hear James's description of the nucleus of the self as ambivalent and fluid. James goes on to describe how, when one looks deeper into this "nucleus" of the personality, there is no essential or substantial center to be found.

> But when I . . . grapple with particulars, coming to the closest possible quarters with the facts, it is difficult for me to detect in the activity any purely spiritual element at all [i.e., any central self]. Whenever my introspective glance succeeds in turning around quickly enough to catch one of these manifestations . . . in the act, all it can ever feel distinctly is some bodily process, for the most part taking place within the head.[3]

The object of James's investigation—a reliable, internal, central, and substantial nucleus of self—turned out to be unfindable and ungraspable. The less we are preoccupied with propping up and maintaining the artifice of self, the closer we are to resting in and acting out of the deep bond between all sentient and insentient life. The path of Yoga helps free us from fixed self-images. Through ongoing opening to the larger world beyond I, me, and mine, we see that I, me, and mine are less solid than we ever thought, and this insight, in turn, loops us back into participation with and feeling for the world, giving us a broader sense of how we are inseparable from the world, and a deeper understanding of what is ultimately real.

Our essential nature does not mean that there is an eternal substance inside me that does not come or go, but rather there is a meaningful connection possible to the experience of life without the superimposition of "me." It is the meaning derived from the intimate relations with life, devoid of self-centeredness, that Hindu terms like *ātman* and *jīva* are pointing at. Wholeness is a multiplicity of things, and by insisting on the clarity of borders and the belief in separateness, we fragment reality into bits and pieces, interrupting any kind of flow or interpenetration.

We always want to know what is behind the personality, within the body, underneath my life. Perhaps, Patañjali suggests, pure awareness (*puruṣa*) is not within or behind this form. Perhaps the masks we wear are all we are and the key is noticing where they stick to us (suffering) and where we can let them transform (freedom). Underneath it all, there is just more and more "underneath"—it never ends. When we read about "the Self" in Indian philosophy, it may seem that there is some internal soul lurking inside the core of my personality. This may be a Judeo-Christian interpretation of the way *self* is used in Indian philosophy, because the self is not at all something that exists in the core of "me"—that would be a dualistic assumption requiring a "me" in relation to "a soul." Rather, the self is a linguistic tool pointing out pure awareness empty of self. Terms like *puruṣa, ātman,* and *jīva* do not refer to individual souls in individual bodies but instead to strategies that humans can use to see nature beyond the fabrication of I, me, and mine. But since language modifies what we "see," it's important to understand why Patañjali is concerned with language and why he doesn't use the term *soul* (*jīva*). By steering clear of metaphysical terms, he points the way toward a language that is conscious of its dualistic constraints.

The base of our life comes down not only to our response to the questions of who and what we are but also to the meaning inherent in intimacy. It's not that being connected with life in the present moment has an inherent meaning but rather that when we are connected with life there is a feeling of life being meaningful. Experience can be meaningful simply by being in it completely. "If life has a base that it stands upon," writes Virginia Woolf,

> then my [life] without a doubt stands upon this memory. It is of lying half asleep, half awake, in bed in the nursery of St. Ives. It is of hearing the waves . . . breaking one, two, one, two behind a yellow blind. It is of hearing the blind draw its little acorn across the floor as the wind blew the blind out. It is of lying and hearing . . . and feeling, it is almost impossible that I should be here.[4]

Who is here? Who reads these words? What falls away when we wake up? Death is the necessity that controls the pattern of life by bringing our experience to a personal conclusion. Facing such a conclusion in each and every moment gives life meaning, not in a personal way and not necessarily with a grand narrative, but simply because profound liberation is available to us when we allow our self-constructed narratives to dismantle and the world to then break in.

We all have memories similar to the one described by Virginia Woolf, when, temporarily, our self-consciousness dissolves and we become lost to the world. The paradox is that when we are lost, we are also found by the world. The world confirms our existence when we no longer need confirmation. Such a grand gesture on the part of the world is the deepest confirmation that we can possibly receive. Sustaining such a transparency of self is the work of Yoga practice. Committing to and refining the fruit of such insight is the ongoing application of the *yamas*.

Yoga offers us the technology—through ethical action and meditative practices—not only to settle the mind and work with habitual energies but also to gain insight into the infinite number of components that make up who we are and what we are. When I look for the boundaries of self, I find myself in the midst of nature. Though the mind's function is to integrate events and help us make meaning through the use of language and boundaries, those boundaries exist only within the mind and dissolve at every opportunity in which we find stillness. We are not in any way separate from anything else. Ocean cliffs get hammered by the wind, falling rain is eventually pulled back into cloud, and the ego is always traumatized by the flux of life. When we are stuck in the framework of a "me" and a "world out there" or a "me" in a body in a world, we alienate our "selves" from the world. Self apart from the world is a mere abstraction because we are not inherently separate from anything. This is why we cultivate stillness: watching the senses and nerves settle over time through quiet breath awareness and steadiness, just like a crane standing in the grass for hours at a time.

Enlightenment means intimacy. We are ready for true awakening when we dissolve the self-made horizons that segregate what is "mine" and what is "yours" and instead stay close to the basic character of ongoing change and nonattachment. As the sun sinks, the stars come out. Realization is the infinite depth of intimacy, where we swim further and further from our names. *Intimacy, freedom,* or even the term *enlightenment* refers to the ability to take care of oneself so that the contracted habits we think of as "me" and "mine" are seen through, and in so doing we open to a larger, more connected reality. It's not that reality changes or that the ego drops away forever. We need an ego. We need a self-image. We need to take care of ourselves and treat the self as sacred. We must care for ourselves in order to truly care for others. What we mean by freedom is that the reactive storyteller inside the mind and the contracted defenses in the vocabulary of the body are seen clearly and thoroughly so that they can be put aside and we can give creative attention to what is going on in and around us.

Rather than conceive of enlightenment as the transcendence of "this" experience, we begin to see how the insight and commitment to our experiences' unfolding in this moment give rise to awakening. Awakening from what? Waking up from a perceived world that pivots around "me."

When I no longer filter my experience through a "me," I can take in much more of what is beyond my personal preference, habits, and knowledge base. In this way I wake up to the world of boundless interrelations. Waking up also presses us to take action. We have a responsibility to respond. One does not have to be engaged in politics to be "engaged." There are many paths of taking action, from staying home and making a garden to writing poems or standing in the way of aggressive development. Waking up to interconnection paired with taking action in the world form the basis of an engaged secular Yoga, a path in tune with these times.

The Bhagavad-Gītā describes how enlightenment is not letting go of the world or renouncing worldly duty or action but rather letting go of clinging to the world through reactivity and attachment to the fruits of one's actions. We let go of our dualistic ways of perceiving and reacting to the world, not worldly life itself.

It is most helpful then to replace the term *enlightenment* with *intimacy* and the word *realization* with *relationship*. Yoga is the restoration of intimacy through body, mind, and heart. By returning us to the body, relational life, and the breath, it brings us into direct relationship with the immediacy of the body and its interactions. The practices restore us to the basic intimate connection we have with all of life. Little by little, we step into our real life, the one that's always been here, because the present always finds us in our bodies, even when we are lost.

The loss of self in yogic terms is the gaining of a more solid ground interconnected not with self-styled ideas of the world but with the reality of a world unmodified by notions of I, me, and mine. The *ahaṅkāra,* the Sanskrit pejorative label for creating narratives of self, unravels through practice when we continually increase our flexibility, not just of the body, but of our modes of perception and our ability to listen. This dissolution of clinging to self-created versions of reality is the key that unlocks the intimacy we call Yoga. The mystical experience is nothing other than the infinite insight into relational existence. I don't suddenly wake up to some eternal place beyond thought where everything is bliss and the world's sorrow and inequality come to an end. I wake up to the way my actions make a difference and to the realization that there are many places where I can serve in order to benefit. I feel that a diligent meditation practice gives rise to the desire to get up and do something. "I" am a fiction that has roots in the world, and when the fiction is seen to be only a narrow version of what we are, we open to a much larger whole.

The "I" is nothing other than a fiction, a world within a world within a fictional world. When one sees that the I is a fiction, the personality begins unraveling into the world without boundaries. And then where is the I to be found? The I is seen to be nothing other than the world itself, playing its unique part but not separate from it. Our everyday practice of Yoga becomes simpler and simpler—open to all states of mind and body: the people we encounter at the store, the water from the tap, our dreams at night, powerful emotions that erupt every now and then. If we open to all of this decisively and without pause, we encounter the world as a part of it. This generates trust and reinforces the truth of being part of a much greater whole. This is no dream, there is no gift to open or heaven to which we must one day ascend; when we arrive in present experience, we come to see that the long carpet of reality is always unrolled. We can't see it when we are looking for only one imagined truth, especially a "truth" that lies outside our lives. The "seeking outward" that often characterizes spiritual endeavor is exactly what obscures the path to intimacy.

Brattleboro, Vermont, 2007

4

The Breath Cycle

We cannot conceive of the birth of anything. There is
only continuation. . . . Look back further and you will
see that you not only exist in your father and mother,
but you also exist in your grandparents and in your
great grandparents. . . . I know in the past I have been
a cloud, a river, and the air. . . . This is the history of life
on earth. We have been gas, sunshine, water, fungi, and
plants. Nothing can be born and also nothing can die.
—THICH NHAT HANH,
The Heart of Understanding

WHEN I LOOK UP at the moon, I can't explain how it came
to be or even how I came to be a man walking on the earth on
this day, at this time, wearing these clothes, and being six feet tall.
Everything I can interact with comes through a multiplicity of tra-
jectories that is governed by forces well beyond my own will and de-
termination. Everything that is human depends on what is not
human. Our true life is the living cosmos as a fluid whole. We slow
down the self-centered turning of mind until we can begin to feel
how the "I" can expand to include everything. The ego does not dis-

solve in spiritual practice; it becomes more imaginative and I until what we thought of as "me" becomes flowering goldenn smooth rocks on the shore, and all other people.

We've all gazed at the moon, we've all listened to profound music, and we've all walked forests at night. These ancient human experiences are Yoga. Yoga is not confined to one culture at one time—it's always been here and continues to be right here.

Yoga is not complete until you practice it. These words are not complete until you read them. One does not finish a piece of music, the audience completes it. Then the critics continue the music in some other form. Likewise the Yoga poses never come to an end. Every morning I return to the breath, and every morning it's brand-new. In some ways my practice has become simpler and simpler because my imagination of what practice is has fallen away. Tending to what's in the midst of my life, beginning with the formality of sitting still every morning, creates grounding that I can't seem to find in other ways.

Tending to the breath and settling the nervous system is the foundation for a responsive social ethic where we take as our first precept: do no harm. While there is no path to a just and peaceful society, there is a way we can all begin taking responsibility for our own actions and compulsions. By committing to a practice of being quiet, waking up the intelligence of the body, and listening and communicating as best I can, I try to embody the teachings of the dharma in everything I do. This kind of commitment always gets me in trouble because I continually fail. Failing becomes the practice.

Turning the cycles of the breath, we begin to trust in something other than the habit drives that keep us caught in false patterns of nourishment. We return to what's important.

The breath cycle has four parts. The inhaling pattern is called *prāṇa* and the exhaling pattern is referred to as *apāna*. *Prāṇa* has the quality of expansion and spreading, and exhaling has a downward and inward pattern. The inhale itself is called *pūraka* and the exhale itself is called *recaka*. As we spin the thread of the breath over longer duration, we also become tuned in to the quality of the pause at the end of the inhale and the pause at the end of an exhale. These pauses, at first, should be very pleasant, much like a rest in a bar of music.

The retention of the breath on the inhale is called *antara kumbhaka*, and the pause at the end of the exhale is called *bāhya kumbhaka*. *Kumbhaka* means "a pot." It precisely refers to the suspension of the *prāṇa* flow. When the *prāṇa* flow is quietly paused, the mind also quiets, because the *prāṇa* and the *citta*—breath and mind—move together as mirrors of one another.

Yoga postures are not an exercise routine in the limited sense. A posture is not something you achieve. The Yoga postures are part of a natural path back to wholeness.

In the *āsana* cycle, we pattern the *vinyāsa* (a series of postures) on this natural, holistic movement. Upward practices happen on the inhale and downward and backward movements always occur on the exhale. In the pause, we release the eyes and the tongue so that there is no tension during the retention. This helps focus the mind and increases the concentration in the Yoga poses. We use breath retentions so that the mind gets very still and so does the breath. The breath actually seems to stop naturally. This helps tone the pelvic diaphragm and provide a solid internal base out of which the mind can rest. This is *samādhi* in physiological language.

In these retentions we refine our patience, and in doing so there is a direct physiological response in the nervous system. The mind and breath work together, and this is vividly apparent in the *prāṇāyāma* practice. The whole universe appears within each breath cycle. The whole universe appears in each moment. The breath brings the universe with it. All the mind patterns show up in these breathing patterns. To us it seems continuous (and there is a continuity in things), but it is a continuity of discrete moments, like a movie. When you watch a movie, it seems continuous, but it is actually a series of independent frames, and each frame is a little bit different from the next frame. Moments of life are like this. They happen so quickly that we don't see the gaps, like a movie. On each one of those discrete moments, the whole universe appears in its entirety. It springs up new—brand-new. The previous moment is gone, and the moments do not impede each other.

In terms of the breath pattern, the inhalation retention begins to feel the same as the exhalation retention. Then we see the one in the other. When the roof of the mouth lifts at the end of an inhale, it takes the reverse shape of the pelvic floor. The inhale includes the exhale and vice versa. Our birth includes our death, and our death includes our birth. One moment of birth is one moment of death. One moment of death is one moment of birth.

We are so restless. This *prāṇāyāma* practice can be so difficult when the mind is agitated. What I love about exploring the retentions is that unlike some forms of *āsana,* the *prāṇāyāma* practice simply doesn't work if the mind is talking along with the breath. Breathing practices bind our attention (*citta*) to the feeling of the breath (*prāṇa*), quieting the distractions of storytelling. Physiology and psychology are two ends of the same stick. You can't work on one without the other.

It is admirable and important to have creative ideas about how to live. Others can't live for you. In these times when we are leaving old institutions and old religious forms, what is becoming most apparent is that we need to practice. A meditation practice that does not begin in and with the body becomes just as intellectualized as anything else. One wandering thought and one distracted breath are no big deal. The problem is they start to link up together until we are lost within ourselves. *Prāṇāyāma* helps set the stage for contemplation in an embodied way. If you set out on the path beyond rules and formulas, *prāṇāyāma* is a good place to start because the practice is visceral and practical. You sit with the breath, move with it, sculpt it. In doing so, you learn about your own mind and stabilize your nervous system.

Zen teacher Zoketsu Norman Fisher describes it this way:

> We don't usually think of spiritual practice as physical, and yet, life, soul, spirit, mind don't exist in the sky, they exist in

association with a body. In Dogen's way of practice, body and mind (or spirit, soul) are one thing, and so to sit—to actually and literally sit down—paying close attention to the body as process, unifying consciousness and breathing with that process until you can enter it wholeheartedly—is to return naturally to what you most truly are.[1]

So Yoga is the power of life beyond and before all definitions. *Prāṇāyāma* tunes us in to this profound vitality, deep intimacy. We are always living out the reality and intimacy of our own lives, although it sometimes happens that we lose sight of this reality. We get caught up in fantasies of the past or of the future, comparing ourselves to others, internalizing expectations. Memory makes things miniature, like a thumbnail for the mind. Practice teaches us how not to get caught by these historical imprints.

So what are we practicing when we practice Yoga? What is the heart of practice? Only you can answer this question. Nobody can practice for you.

Athens, Greece, 2007

5

The Object of Meditation

If from moment to moment your mind dwells on what
is and then drops it effortlessly at once, the mind becomes no-mind, full of peace.
—VAŚIṢṬHA, *Yoga Vasiṣṭha*

ONE OF THE PRACTICES Patañjali is very clear about is that
if one does not choose an object of meditation, the mind simply wanders into and through its favorite grooves.[1] If you've ever
tried to sit still and simply notice what's happening, it becomes clear
that the momentum of the mind's habits take over until we are sky-
flighting every which way. Patañjali offers us some guidelines in his
textbook, the *Yoga-Sūtra:*

3.1. Concentration locks attention on one single area.
3.2. When the attention settles into the object completely, the entire perceptual flow becomes aligned with that object.
3.3. When only the essential nature of the object shines forth, as if
formless, subject and object dissolve and intimacy arises.
3.4. These three consecutive practices—concentration, attention
settling, and intimacy—compose the perfect discipline of
awareness.

3.5. Once the attention is stabilized in this way, wisdom dawns.

3.6. Cultivating stable awareness in service of intimacy occurs in these stages.

3.7. These three practices (*dhāraṇā, dhyāna, samādhi*) are much more internal and quiet than the preceding practices (of *yama, niyama, āsana, prāṇāyāma, pratyāhāra*).[2]

We live in an attention-deficit society. Our attention is always getting trapped by advertising, the Internet, traffic, and shopping. In the practice Patañjali describes, our attention is trained in stages so that it can hold the object in view for a longer and longer time. If the object is the breath, we can stay with the feeling of inhaling and exhaling without much distraction for a long period of time. This is called *dhāraṇā*. Then we find the mind eventually settles and the object (the breath) also settles. This is called *dhyāna*. Eventually the observer who is telling the mind that everything is settling completely falls away, as does language. Then there is a deep stillness where we feel that we are simply part of a much greater whole. I've translated this term (*samādhi*) as "intimacy" so as to reflect the felt sense of this experience. But *samādhi* is temporary. You can't hold on to it.

One of the interesting things about choosing the breath as an object of meditation is that unlike other meditation objects, it does not instill much craving, desire, or an increase of stimulus. When you choose a mantra, for example, the more you focus on the sound or meaning of it, the clearer it becomes—it becomes quite vivid. But with the breath, the more you focus on the feeling and texture of the movement of inhaling and exhaling, the more subtle and gentle and shallow it becomes.

Because the breath monitors the state of the nervous system, and because the quality of the nerves determines the quality of our attention, a constant feedback loop is created. The breath regulates the body, which in turn regulates the mind, which in turn determines the quality of attention on the breath.

The longer we sustain attention on the breath, the softer it gets.

But if we are distracted after some time, immediately the breath be comes coarse again. This is actually helpful: if the breath remained subtle, it would be hard to locate. So when you are caught in commentary or laxity, your breath becomes coarse and then easy to connect with.

In the Yoga postures, we are always making sure the background of every pose has the quality of both *sthirā* and *sukha,* steadiness and ease. This means that we continually follow this feedback loop between the *prāṇa* and the *citta,* the energy in the breath/body and the movement of consciousness. If there is too much effort in the pose, the breath becomes agitated and the nerves hinder the movement of the muscles, fascia, and somatic layers of the pose. These various strands all penetrate one another, but it's easiest to keep impeccable awareness on the quality of the breath.

Yoga posture sequences are patterned on the inherent rhythms of inhaling and exhaling. The postures are not just laid down on top of the breath patterns but are actually animated and sustained by them. Because the inhaling breath is conducive to upward and outward actions (*prāṇa*), and the exhaling breath conducive to backward and downward patterns (*apāna*), we have a framework on which to observe the movements of the mind. When we feel the breathing pattern as the foundation of each Yoga pose, we can begin to watch how the mind moves and relates to the different patterns of sensation that coincide with these posture sequences.

Each set of postures sets up sensation patterns out of which the mind also creates patterns of thought, image, story, and association. Usually the patterns swing between attachment (*rāga*) and aversion (*dveṣa*) to the feeling tone of the pose. When the mind enters the stream of the pose, we find that there is movement but the mind remains relatively stable, relatively still. When the mind is still, it does not create categories and preferences. Then the breath can move through the rivers of the body (*nāḍīs*) uninterrupted. When distraction settles, we can tune in to the pathways of energy that open as the breath steadies in the pattern of the pose. Again, when we get distracted, the breath becomes coarse. When the breath is coarse, the mind moves out into the more superficial layers of the *āsana*. When the breath is even and steady and the postures are linked within the breath cycle, the mind is free to investigate and notice without getting stuck in any one place. This is the internal form of Yoga, the internal tradition of the Yoga *āsana*.

In the *Yoga-Sūtra,* Patañjali states clearly that the Yoga posture should be accompanied by the loosening of tension (*prayatna*), which gives rise to the indivisibility of the body and the infinite universe.[3]

There is no separation. The key to the coalescence (*samāpatti*) of this *samādhi* (intimacy) is that the background of the practice is rooted in relaxation. When the mind is at ease, the *prāṇa* is at ease. When we develop one-pointed concentration, the whole background has to be at ease. When we practice deep Yoga poses, the eyes and face must be at ease.

Without the background of ease, a muscle contraction takes over. Effort must relax for intimacy to appear. "[Intimacy] occurs," declares Patañjali, "when all effort relaxes and coalescence arises, revealing that the body and the natural world are indivisible."[4]

The combination of settling the body energies through *āsana* and *prāṇāyāma* sets the stage for deeper levels of meditative quietude to appear. As concentration coalesces in the following limbs of concentration and meditation, we begin to see clearly how our perceptions color all of our interactions with life. This helps us look at the projector rather than at what is projected. It helps us withdraw our ideas about others and ourselves. It is a very practical process. Then we will be better prepared to flow with what is happening, to act creatively. You don't have to be a yogi or a Buddhist or adopt a new belief system. Sitting quietly, wordlessly, can make it a habit—this awareness that our words for the world are not the same as what's really out there. When frequently reinforced, this understanding will cast light on all of our interactions in and as life. All of our interactions will then constitute practice. This is freedom. Then we can recognize the way we get hooked, the way we hook others, the way the hook operates. Leonard Cohen sums this up clearly:

> So I must say it quickly:
> Whoever is in your life,
> Those who harm you,
> Those who help you;
> Those whom you know
> And those whom you do not know—
> Let them off the hook,
> Help them off the hook.
> Recognize the hook.
> You are listening to Radio Resistance.[5]

Montreal, Quebec, 2007

PART TWO

Body, Mind, and the Natural World

6

The Quality of Flow

self nature that is no nature . . .
far beyond mere doctrine.
—HAKUIN ZENJI, "SONG OF ZAZEN"

WHILE FOLLOWING the curving trails alongside the Elbow
River in Calgary, Alberta, I stop every few minutes to listen
to the rippling sounds of moving water. There is a large steel and copper bridge that crosses the river, and in relation to the movement of
water, the bridge seems completely still. Immediately my mind creates two opposing categories: movement and stillness.

But when I begin walking along the bridge that crosses the rushing waters, the braided copper cables shift. The wooden planks creak,
and the bridge moves and sways subtly. In relationship to the water
that I see between the wooden foot planks, the bridge is moving and
the water is still. In relation to the land, the bridge is flowing. The
bridge now has the quality of water.

Once I cross the bridge and arrive on dry land, I follow the path
that curves left and down toward the shore. The path is more like an
unfinished trail of trampled grasses and worn river rocks. The trail is
also changing. From the bridge, my mind associated the trail with
solid earth in opposition to the flowing water. But because the trail is

created by dogs and humans and beavers making their way to the river, it too is changing, it too has the quality of flow. The river, the bridge, and the trail: all flow.

The Yoga postures I practiced before my walk—the backbends (called bridge pose)—also have the quality of water. Animated by the breath, the pose is never complete. It shifts and moves and flows not just into other postures but within itself as well.

Everything has this quality of flow. Letters flow to form words, and the meaning of these words as I speak and write them will flow into meaning for you, the listener or reader. Listening to this talk or reading it on paper reminds us that the sentence is not finished when it is articulated; it continues its life in your mind, the one listening.

A beaver pokes its head out of the stream and then drops into the subcurrent of the river and swims upstream. Though the water rushes downward to the south, the beaver catches the opposite current, only one meter deep, and without effort floats upstream. Our ideas of stillness and movement, liquidity and solidity, appear to be the truth of how things are. But when we quiet the mind and look clearly, there is another truth below our conceptual thoughts, and it's to *this* that Yoga orients us.

Yoga, defined as intimacy or basic union, reminds us that if everything is connected to everything else, we must confront the illusion that people are free to exploit nature and move in society in ways that exploit others. Yogic ethics nurture nature while nurturing people as well. How can we replace helplessness and apathy with an empowering social vision, practical psychological tools, and an articulate ecological perspective?

From Chernobyl to the Gulf of Mexico oil spill, depletion is interlinked with social imbalance in ways never before experienced on this planet. Grasses, humans, animals, and rivers cannot be repaired or controlled by parts of a machine. Mind is not separate from body either: the scent of a flower cannot be separated from the sight of a flower. Life is psychosomatic, relational, and inherently united.

The vortex in a stream is a structure that is created out of the swirling gravitational movement of water. All living things are flowing structures like this. Our identity, sexuality, economics, and relations are all temporary and flexible. One of the aspects of practicing in the context of community (*sangha*) that I've deeply appreciated is the way people can relate to one another with less competitiveness, less egoic strategizing. With a focus on practice and expressing this practice in everyday situations, we can dismantle the prominence of individual egos pursuing individual ends, replacing it with a more inclusive and community-based understanding. Watch people change over time: it's interesting to notice how elastic our egoic habits are and also how spiritual practice in the context of *sangha* supports care for others.

Let us declare a peace with the natural world, where all of our activities support biodiversity and cultural diversity. Let's establish a thoughtful, caring, and tender way of being in and of the world. This ethic respects the *prāṇa* of everyday life: bird *prāṇa*, human *prāṇa*, forest *prāṇa*, river *prāṇa*. The winds (*prāṇa vāyu*) are everywhere and in everything, sustaining every human perception, breath, and thought. If there were such a thing as a spiritual ecology, we might be able to listen to the imbalance of *prāṇa* and wonder how we can help bring the great winds of life back into balance.

Calgary, Alberta, 2008

7

Organizing in the Natural World

For life in the present there is no death. Death is not an
event in life. It is not a fact in the world. Our life is endless, in just the same way that our field of vision has no
boundaries.
—WITTGENSTEIN, *Tractatus*
Logico-Philosophicus

WHAT DOES IT MEAN that our field of vision has no
boundaries? I look into a river and see fish and stones and
moss and the reflection of the sky and birds and humans. In the river
there is nothing other than everything. It's a cold winter day, and my
son wanted to have a long bath before school this morning. He said
the water was just "really hot snow." Before it can put an end to its
own elaborations, the mind creates the world out of boundaryless-
ness. Such union is the basis for the mind-body-world to begin with.
These words are just the words of winter. Winter writes itself on the
branches and grasses. But when I am in stillness, I can't find the line
between those branches and the limbs of my body.

Although a person is not *exactly* water and earth and air and fire,
we are also not separate from those elements either. We are not sepa-

rate or identical to the elements. If we search for any one thing we can pinpoint as objectively real—one thing we really depend on for our existence—we will fail. We can't land on one defining characteristic.

The Yoga that precedes "this" and "that," "mind" and "body," is percolating through your every movement today—every thought, word, and deed. Everything you think and feel and do is temporary. Everything you see and hear is passing away. This reminder of death in life is following each and every one of us. A simple and gentle reminder but relentless nevertheless: don't drift. Don't squander your life.

Mind is not just a human function or organ but the natural condition of living systems. Wherever there is life there is mind. Biological systems, from embryos to social insects, get tremendous mileage by using vast numbers of easy-to-find, unreliable components to achieve complex evolutions reliably. One year after a forest fire, the land is itself on fire—teeming with insects and other breathing creatures.

Mind is always organizing. We humans classify the raw data of our experience by giving it name and form. Mind is what puts name and form together. When we can see that our mind is a kind of synthesizer, we can step back and watch the choices that our minds make moment to moment. The greatest freedom we have is being able to clearly see that in any given context, we have choice. We can decide what kind of attention and attitude we bring to the object showing up here and now. And it can change. This life-and-death cycle of thoughts and attitudes reminds us that choice is always present. There is immense freedom in choice. How we pay attention is a liberating resource.

Death happens in life: it's in your breath cycle, the blink of your eye, the collapse of your favorite ideas, the loss of someone close to you. I sat with my uncle Ian, my closest friend, for the hours leading up to his death. Longer and longer exhales, with longer and longer pauses between inhales, eventually gave way to his passing. He was quiet and at ease. In his last moments I fell in love with him again and again. His eyes were closing and he had nothing to say.

When I walked out of the hospital two hours later, the street was bustling with life. Ambulances pulling up to the emergency doors, families leaving the hospital with newborn babies, streetcars full of students on their way to the university. Everywhere I walked for the next few hours seemed so alive and precious. Death in life reminds us not just that our lives are structured by death but that death is occurring in each and every movement. The movement of thoughts, breathing, feeling, perception, walking, and talking are all transient phenomena. I missed my uncle, but I was also merged with the ongoing flow of life happening in and around me. Life unfolding includes death—this is city dharma, birth dharma, death dharma, streetcar dharma—the interpenetration of death in life and life structured by death.

Systems are patterns of relationships that are organized. They have "rules" that govern their behavior. One such rule is impermanence. But if you search life for death, you can't find it. And if you search the death experience for life, it's also invisible. Look closely though: you can find both simultaneously. There is life in death as there is death in life. The pattern of organization is not imposed from outside but "comes with" the system at the moment of creation. It is the system itself that organizes itself around some sort of operating principle. The mind is always trying to get outside the system in order to know the operating principle. This is the birth of religion. As we try to get larger than the physical (metaphysical), we create stories that give us a sense of permanence in a highly contingent world. The bird chirps and I have endless ideas about how and why: it might be chirping. But can I investigate the bird chirping with my whole body? *Who* hears the chirp?

This morning a fish brushed my leg as I walked upstream from the bridge at Machar-Strong boundary road. As the fish touched my leg, I wondered if "leg" and "fish" organized that experience any differently. The legs, perhaps like the fish as well, each have their own way of having that experience. I like to make stories and even exaggerate, as if the fish were coming to tell me something or that my leg was in the way of its route home to its lover. And then I began to wonder about the biological importance of water, how the land, streams, and seas are all connected. How my daily habits and consumer choices affect aquatic life. Who speaks for the fish?

When this vastness appears to me—when it appears in general—it can only appear like this. It can only appear through my body, my life, my joys, my faults. Every moment includes exactly everything without limit. My self-expression is not my own. Every life and every moment of every life in every place is the only truth of existence right now. Reality is unnameable and immeasurable, but at the same time it manifests as you and me. When we die, so too will this uniqueness. Yoga practice is not a mystery—it is recalling who we really are.

When the selfless mode of perception—what we call nondualism, or Yoga—is sustained, it comes with a feeling of connectedness and deep relationship with all of life. It gives us energy. It is the ongoing refinement and inclusion of these insights into the reality and grime of life that compel me to choose a life of teaching. For all of us, this wider understanding of Yoga brings into focus the importance of formal and informal practice and the central role of relationship in spiritual life. We see that the locus of connectedness in our lives is visceral and not mental. Our body is a living landscape, and our mind is a part of this landscape, with a continuity extending in every direction. If we all share in the ebb and flow of causality (karma), our actions of body, speech, and mind become our most creative expression of interconnectedness.

Each aspect of this pathless path involves refining our modes of perception and our ways of acting. Yoga begins and culminates in relationship. The mystical experience—the insight that wakes us up—is nothing other than seeing into the nature of the present moment free from "adding anything," free from human preference and the habits of dualistic perception.

The search for meaning in life and the search for a way to be fully alive in life are inseparable. We can't separate our feelings about the world from our deepest feelings about ourselves. Patañjali articulates the way action in the world—whether that action is given the name spirituality, ethics, or psychology—begins in the present moment through choices that we make.

Guelph, Ontario, 2008

8

Not Closing Our Eyes

The world we have made as a result of the level of thinking we have done thus far creates problems we cannot
solve at the same level we created them.
—ATTRIBUTED TO ALBERT EINSTEIN

W E CANNOT ESCAPE our lives. The world as experienced
in your body right now—your mind as it observes, then
contributes to the parade of thinking as you read these words—
cannot be exchanged for the experience of another. It feels as though
I am having my own unique thoughts and feelings and you are experiencing yours. Because we can't surgically separate the thoughts you
are having right now from the colors of this room or the icebergs that
silently glide thousands of miles north and south of here, everything
you experience right now is one. Everything in the world is the
ground of our life. Though your thoughts happen in unique configu-
rations because of your past, your conditioning, and your DNA, it's
also interesting to see that these thoughts are all a process of the great
mind, the transpersonal, interpersonal world in mind.

When I first started practicing Yoga, I thought the practice would
lead to a cessation of thinking altogether. I also imagined that I'd be
able to somehow leave my body, especially since my body was in pain.

It was surprising when I began to realize that the practice of sequential Yoga postures, combined with full breathing and the stillness of meditation, actually stabilized the chattering of my mind and body long enough so there was room for my more difficult and challenging habitual drives to arise. What was left when my mind became almost still was not quietude but discomfort—and the discomfort certainly didn't feel like oneness.

One of the ideas that I had about perception was that I could somehow have such pure attention that my human perspective could dissolve altogether. I hoped I could float above my body so that I could witness experience but not partake of it. Of course it was easy to become still enough that my name and past and gender dissolved for a time. At least, it took a backseat to the tree and the snow and the sound of the ice breaking up. I imagined I could just swim away from my name. When this happened I conceived that this was momentary *samādhi*. In actual fact, it would always lead to the arising of intense loneliness and disquiet. Was there any way, I wondered, that I could move through the world without putting human handprints all over it? Could I find in myself a kind of protected neutrality, untouched by dramatic feelings and internal conflict? Was there a way out?

One day on retreat I had finished *āsana* practice, and the wind was blowing against the meditation room as the rain clouds moved dramatically overhead. The sky looked like it was filled with heavy black party streamers. I was on an island in the Pacific Northwest, and the birds had come in from the ocean to rest on the windowsills. I sat still and looked at the birds sitting by the window, and I was filled with anxiety. I was taken back to my new home at six years old. . . .

The bay window leans out over our front yard. I sit in the window seat and look into the red Japanese maples that brush against the front of our house. It smells like vinegar and newsprint. The bus goes by, and then it's silent again. I see the reflection of my mother, behind me, in the glass, and as in a dream in which you try to speak but your voice is muted, I try to make contact with her, but only her reflection remains. I feel incredibly lonely. My mother, the one I most need, is unfindable. No contact. There she is in the dark glass, and all I can do is touch her image with my eye. Not her body, not her skin, not her words. She could not listen. She could not hear me. I can't recall any other details. I might even have fallen asleep.

As I sat on retreat looking at the glass windows, my body was filled with these old emotions, memories of loss and disconnection. But there was nowhere to go. Just this solitary room on a desolate island on the Pacific coast. As the clouds collected outside, I felt my body was going to explode, but I had nowhere to go. Absorbed by this past-present pain, I sat and sat until I could feel the floor, the ground, and the breath. And as I sat, the eruption of anxiety and loneliness slowly began to pass, like the clouds overhead. With sudden choreography and a loud whoosh against the window, the birds took off back toward the ocean. The storm had passed.

So much of our discontent has to do with distrust of our body knowledge, mistaking what is transient as permanent. On this morning of the retreat I described, the walls and the floor and the breath became an intuitive mother-body support, holding me without saying a word. I was five and six and seven and ten, and I was also thirty, allowing the envelope of the sky, the birds, and memory to hold me together. Ambivalent memories of unavailability and cancellation were held together by stillness with such a lasting effect that over the hours that passed, I felt cleaned out and alive.

We all have attacking or unwanted figures in our memories, both physically and emotionally. And as the shaft of awareness drops down lower and lower, as the breath draws deeper into the core of the body, these competing and unwanted emotions arise. The practice teaches us how to open to these experiences. Equanimity (*upekṣā*) is not a silent witnessing of our psychic lives but an opening toward *what is*. And these difficult emotions are not distractions or impingements on the meditative path. They are the very path itself.

Our lives all take a unique shape, like grain in wood, veined stones, codes of DNA. Opening to the way these past impressions (*vāsana*) appear in the body-mind (*saṃskāra*) and emerge into awareness as specific symptoms (*granthi*) is the heart of Yoga, the path of intimacy. This is how we embrace the heart of the world. Taking care of ourselves, we take care of one another. One hand will always wash the other.

Meditation practices are essential for realizing this level of intimacy because through stillness we learn that underneath the surface distractions of consciousness in body and mind, there is a visceral sense of connectedness with all of life. At first this feels like connection to a mood or a thought, but over time we begin to see that what we think of as our character or even our truest self is, in fact, the entire world. With such a realization, how can we not respond with kindness and action?

Sometimes compassion begins as a very small drop, like the way white skeins of mist drift across the sky from nowhere. We are so much more empathic when the mind is not skittish, when we are not unhappy with ourselves. I stood looking up at a tree yesterday trying to see if it was the same green as my sweater. I noticed how quiet it was, and so I closed my eyes and just stood there. Suddenly a crow darted out from a tangle of shadow, startling my eyes open, and I saw its glassy eyes. That bird had been there the whole time. Maybe compassion is mixed in with everything too.

Compassion (*karuṇā*) occurs when we move with equanimity right to the edge of violence. It's relatively easy to find equanimity through formal meditation practice and time on retreat. But the heart of nonviolence practice occurs right at the edge of violence. We need to bring attentiveness to the times when anger is building in us, or we are caught in compulsions that are turning us inside out. Sometimes we need to pause and wait. And this open waiting is receptive action, an action without the stress and compulsion of reactivity. Intimacy occurs right at this edge of conflict. We bring up difficulties with our friends, we talk about how we feel, we challenge one another when we are having difficulty. Politically it means stepping up for what we believe in, protecting those who cannot speak up, not closing our eyes.

Deep Yoga is not the small feeling of interconnectedness we might feel lying in corpse pose at the end of a Yoga class—it is moving into the frayed territory where we are most uncomfortable. Challenging a friend or colleague in an unsatisfying personal relation, or talking to your teenager about something that may be uncomfortable for you both—these are acts of Yoga, acts of intimacy that characterize a practice activated in our everyday lives.

Renunciation is like undressing all the fear and resistance that characterize defensiveness so that we can enter into life without reservation. The anorexic speaks up about her preoccupation with food; the shy introvert tells her lover how hard it is for her to express herself; the busy lawyer stays home for the weekend and plays with his children. Our symptoms are frozen scenes wanting to be thawed, needing to come to life. In my early years studying Yoga I was also a student of psychoanalysis, reading Patañjali and Freud side by side. I was struck by the way Freud saw the psychological symptoms in his patients as being rooted in both mind and body. He made little distinction between pain in the body and its manifestation in the emotions and imagination. In his *Studies on Hysteria* (1893),[1] Sigmund Freud recognized that people were not telling him (and themselves) the whole story. He asked his patients to lie down and relax and see what comes to mind. He would sit by the couch and listen "with evenly hovering attention"[2] in such a way that the silent listening of the doctor and the verbal expression of the patient meshed, revealing repetitive patterns that would be discussed and explored. This would lift inhibition.

In our Yoga practices at Centre of Gravity we do a lot of partner exercises. I also meet students one-on-one in order to talk together about what is happening in their practice, their life. Without this kind of challenge of self-expression, our inner world can be avoided and our insights can remain private and inactivated in daily life. What a relief it is to reveal our secrets.

Freud was so interested in the way we make slips—a word is spoken in relaxed awareness before we realize it has slipped out. But it can't be erased. The cure for Freud was not just putting things into words but challenging the patient to find his or her *own* words. In the context of relationship, the patient can begin to digest and metabolize what was previously frozen through repression. As we express ourselves we shape our lives in new and sometimes unexpected ways. Behind words is the silence that supports honesty and self-reflection. These two together—silence and expression—form the medium of creative human expression.[3]

When we conceive of "waking up" as transcendence, we take *disjunction* as the primary assumption. When we conceive of enlightenment as a horizontal recognition of intimacy, we take *continuity* as a primary focus. Instead of projecting heaven forward in time and up in space, we can imagine heaven as the topography of our relational lives. Life can be felt as interdependent, without mythic and transcendental principles to explain how it works. Can we imagine transcendence as a process that brings us into the body, into relationship, and into self-expression, rather than up and away? Can we return to awareness the old emotions, pains, memories, and inadequacies we've been filing away deep in memory?

Can these disparate parts of ourselves communicate with one another? Can we allow the unbearable to unfold and shake our foundations until it becomes silence once again? Even when we don't listen, the silent song of the world is coursing through life. And life is one giant, open, looping communication pathway.

Everyone communicates: the sparrow with the blue jay, the ants with one another, the queen bee and her workers, the woman at her doorstep thanking the mailman. The quality of this communication is what's key. Language is not just a human invention—neither is poetry nor song. Walk through a forest and listen to the gossip. In a culture so focused on production and consumption and the singular idol of monetary currency, we are quickly losing not just the wild world of birds and bees and forests but also the myriad forms of language that keep us humans vital and alive.

When we get stuck in our internal commentary or in chronic moods, it becomes hard to tune in to the flow of expression that marks healthy relations. Over time we end up feeling isolated and alone. Yoga asks you to pour yourself out, just like the sun.

When we think of our emotions ecologically, as parts of a complex and dynamic mind-body system, we realize that even anger and distress have a valid place. If life needs to be lived in communion with every other form of life that also wants to live, then nothing should be left out.

Los Angeles, 2007

9

Ontario Snow Lineage

Xiushan said, "What can you do about the world?"
Dizang said, "What do you call the world?"
—*Book of Serenity*, CASE 12

WE'VE BEEN ON retreat for only two days now, and the impact of the snow crystallizes each and every moment. I love the sound of walking in the snow. Imagine measuring time by listening to snow falling. Some mornings, the wall, both imaginary and literal, that separates me from snow feels less than paper thin. The walls in this meditation hall are thin, and in this wonderful winter retreat environment so are the mind-erected walls. If I could maintain such a delicate state of mind, there would be no use for words any longer. There would be no "any longer." Sometimes without words everything seems possible. Does anyone else feel this way?

The snow is so supportive of our practice. Several years ago I drove out to the forests and rivers in northern Ontario to return to the basic questions that motivated my spiritual quest in the first place: How do I live a life in the face of impermanence and a pervasive sense of suffering and imbalance not just in human terms but across the spectrum of life? What can I do in the world? How do I find meaning and beauty even when I know that human interference is rapidly destroying the delicate and beautiful balance of the natural world? The rivers are ill, the cities polluted, the urban sky almost always a shade of brown. I came to this northern land on a kind of sabbatical or retreat. Every good idea eventually becomes a bad idea. Every solution eventually becomes stale. For example, I'm enjoying fatherhood and teaching and writing, but I've needed a short break to reconsider what I'm doing. Maybe retreat is a way of leaving behind the answers I've found in the past several years through practice and research and teaching.

It was in this cold northern forest that I discovered Yoga, and so I've returned to begin taking what I've discovered apart to reconsider the basic existential dilemmas of being alive in a life structured by death. I'm lucky my son's mother can look after him for a while so that I can visit the white land. Snow supports this endeavor through its relentless beauty and stillness. Snow changes while also being still. And it falls so silently. Snow changes the way I experience myself.

There is a need in our Western culture, both personally and socially, for another way of looking at the world that is much more complete, satisfying, and sharp in its ability to address certain questions in our lives that we don't find answers for in our own traditions. This is snow Yoga, the Ontario lineage. The snow breaks up the infinite wallpaper that we call mind. Or, putting it another way, our attentiveness to the snow shows us we have choice in the way we pay attention. As we give our attention fully to any one thing, attentiveness derails the old tracks of the binary mind and opens us up to many more options. Freedom has everything to do with the choice that opens through attentiveness. Attentiveness disrupts craving and rejection, two sides of the coin that give rise to a one-track mind. While we will never overcome suffering once and for all, we can certainly bring craving to an end. Bringing the scattered mind into attentiveness is the beginning of freedom, and it comes by yoking attention to whatever is presenting itself in that moment.

When you don't name them, snow walking and snow melting are *samādhi*. *Samādhi* is the integration of attention and what's happening in present experience. (Somehow I need to share with you what my experience is and has been, through words and sentences, and in so doing, stay connected to what my experience was then and is now. Yet the past is gone! I am well aware of the paradox. Speaking of the past now becomes a retrospective mindfulness practice.) The breath, the air in the pine forest, and the spaces between the vertebrae intermingle with every other space, every clearing, every emptiness. The different patches of blue in the thick dense sky, the endless trickling of the melting ice in the eaves trough. The robust wind and the spider trapped between two old boards. This old house shivers through the winter.

It takes time for the mind and body to settle into stillness. Sometimes when I am in a Yoga posture, I give attention to the breath and wait and wait. I wait for the nerves, all those little synapses, to register the grounding limbs and the uplifting breath. It takes time for the body to fully receive the breath, the pattern of the posture, the calmness available in attentiveness. It takes time before we can stay with the in breath and out breath without much distraction. Returning to the breath is a process, like our hands learning the feel of new tools. The natural world of breathing and attentiveness resists being absorbed into the television of the mind.

Awareness is a long beautiful arc that at once encompasses and witnesses everything in movement. But *witness* is simply a word. It's not a very good choice anyway, because in the experience of deep sitting practice, "the witness" falls away, as do all categories and oppositions, revealing the universe as infinite and indivisible.

The unshakable sanity that comes from the wellspring of silence returns us to our selves—and in no way is that separate from the ongoing flux of the natural world. In a moment, the universe is both intimate and universal. What could be more quietly subversive?

In the third line of the *Yoga-Sūtra,* Patañjali reminds us that our basic nature is the nature of everything, although this insight is concealed by misidentifying with the endless distractions of our thoughts.

"When all fluctuations in the mind are seen as only fluctuations of mind, the seer dwells in its own form."[1] As long as we continue to misidentify with the distractions, calling them "I," "me," "mine," or "the truth," we take the form of those fluctuations rather than engagement with what actually is. Through discriminative awareness (*viveka-khyāti*) we can begin to plant positive states of mind where negative states previously lived. Some of the most inspiring practitioners are the ones I know whose lives are filled with extraordinary problems. Pain, loss, confusion, and illness are all part of what it costs to be human. All the components necessary for spiritual life are grounded in the here and now. Nothing is hidden.

So if nothing is hidden, transcendence is a means of waking up to the fact that we are already home. We allow our lives to be dominated by the assumption that life is a mystery that must be uncovered. Why do we feel that the answer to the great questions of life can only be accessed by looking into some secret chamber? Perhaps the more time we spend in the snow, the more we'll see how life is not hidden. Letting go in meditation practice shows us how we've traded in all of these mysteries for explanations and concepts that don't always give life meaning and value. It's cold out today, and the surface of the snow is filled with little craters. This natural beauty is far beyond theology. If you're like me and you keep falling for the mental world of symbols, spend some time entering the shape of the snow, the frozen swamp, icicles on rocks reflecting back to us.

Our distractions are a smoke screen, and we forget that seeing, like being, is not a "self" activity at all. When the bustling modifications of thought become still, when the smoke clears, awareness and the phenomenal world seem interdependent but not quite the same. At first, awareness can be described as unchanging. But when we step even beyond that, the felt experience is one of complete alignment: enmeshment *in* and *of* and *as* everything. *Samādhi* is like being initiated into the earth once again.

After many years of studying Yoga philosophy in depth and practicing in a disciplined and exacting way, I started to feel that the old texts and the nuanced discourses had little to say about the inevitable paragons of conflict in my life. They were not relevant to the imbalances in the natural and economic world around me. I felt the need to take what I had learned and put it to work in every area of life, not just my personal activity. How can we bomb people on the other side of the ocean and continue to believe we live in a free and democratic world? I just can't think of myself as being apolitical. I can't even imagine the Buddha as someone who was not immersed in the social and cultural and political dilemmas of his time. Jesus was a man committed to his economic situation as well. Ideas of a life outside the particularities of one's layered activity is too idealistic for me. It makes no sense. When we look into the layers of our conditioning, we find the conditioning of our culture as well, with all of its biases and spins. Spiritual practice must deal with these very real issues as well.

Instead of continuing to teach Yoga texts in a line-by-line manner, chanting syllables and breaking down the ancient commentaries and etymological details, I began challenging myself and my students to contemplate the way the teaching could come alive in the most obscure places. How, for example, can teachings of concentration be put to work in our relational lives? What role does ethics play in our psychological well-being?

Yoga teachings are not a response to life that stand apart from its movement. Yoga is a living question that continually points its practitioner back toward his or her own life, back into the body, straight into community. An ongoing practice recognizes that there is a transcendent mystery beyond the techniques that a practice employs. Awakening is not the end result of a systematized process. Reawakening love and intimacy for one's self and beyond requires practice. This is not because love is something far away from us but because we forget. We forget that intimacy is near. We forget how to relax with others. We forget we are whole. Realization is a kind of remembering rather than an achievement or virtuosic accomplishment. Practice awakens the dormant and often invisible interiors of mind, body, and heart in order to establish a more tender, responsive, creative, and active self.

The quiet snow reinvigorates my desire to point out where we all get stuck in comfort and blindness. More so, the quiet time in the snow fills me again with the energy required to go back into the public world and talk about the value of snow and creative action. The luminosity of the natural and wild restores me to my senses. With unrushed insight and keen eyes, we can all feel utterly at ease even though there is much work ahead.

Northern Ontario, 2005

10

Liberation

The greatest poverty is not to live
In a physical world
—WALLACE STEVENS,
"ESTHETIQUE DU MAL," XV

As I WALKED down to the building this evening through the dappled light and snow, I caught the first shadows of the eclipse that is going on tonight. The origin of the word *mokṣa*, which we use to describe enlightenment or awakening, has its roots in the symbolism of an eclipse. *Mokṣa*, etymologically, refers to the last phase of an eclipse where as one body begins to move out of the way of the other, the latter shines forth. This evening, the shadow of the earth crossed in front of the moon, but as soon as the shadow receded, the moon shone once again.

I like this understanding of *mokṣa* much more than the term *enlightenment*. When we use the term *enlightenment,* it's fraught with too much cultural interpretation. It obscures what it feels like as we gradually, and sometimes suddenly, recognize the way our minds are capped with and stained by our old blinding habits. When we describe this process as waking up, it more accurately reflects the gradual process of finding freedom from the self-imposed constraints that bog us down and reinforce feelings of separation and lack. Awakening is a process of waking up rather than of finding a permanent and eternal state of mind. Just as the eclipsed moon is stained by the shadow of the earth as it slowly crosses between the sun and the moon, awakening can happen and then be overshadowed by everyday, earthly existence. But practice allows it to shine forth again, as Patañjali says, "lifting the veil revealing the mind's inherent luminosity."[1]

If we think of *mokṣa* as moving up and out of this body or the cessation of all thinking or the end of all relations, enlightenment becomes an impossible and unhealthy vertical achievement. It's all about "me," a rocket blasting off the planet's crust trying to get out of here in any way possible. The upward and outward urge misses this experience of the mind and body completely because it's an attempt to get beyond it. But even if we flew past the moon and millions of years and orbits away from here, we would be no closer to "it" than we are now. Meanwhile, here we are, in bodies, in clothes, experiencing, or encountering, or entangled with one another. There is nothing so precious and so beautiful.

Since the earliest days of our human history, we've been narrating huge arcing stories to give meaning to our place here. Where do we go when we die? We've never come up with an ultimately satisfying response, so would it be too much to ask that we just put that question aside? Does it not distract us from what's going on here and now? The human life is spent in pursuit of a total visionary understanding of where we are heading and what we can secure for ourselves in the future. What if we change the direction of these stories so that life is not ascending anywhere? Why push this vague notion of "me" in the future so high in our imagination? When you pay close attention to your inhalation materializing and coming to a silent pause, and then the exhalation trailing down into the lower abdomen and eventually coming to a still point, you begin to see that you are leaving these stories behind, leaving yourself behind, every moment of life. In fact, there are no moments, there is no present, there is not such a grip on time. When the resolute mind lightens up, it flows into and out of the world quite lightly. The other extreme is a determined and complete vision of an absolute that must exist, and if it does not, "my practice is failing." This is an impossible extreme.

In the face of such a stark reality, we want to flee into the Absolute, flee into our stories of transcendence and the eternal. A modern, secular Yoga will have none of that. You live not by securing yourself *against* impermanence but by finding yourself *as* impermanence. We live by pouring ourselves out. In retrospect we might conceive of this as "self-realization," but in the experience, *mokṣa* is just the unveiling of intimacy. Freud and Heidegger and Kierkegaard and Samuel Beckett were all terrified of the absence of storytelling. They thought of it as some kind of void or abyss.[2] I'm not sure if the notion of a void is really such a negative thing. We are always living a dying life. Anyone working with the breathing body day in and day out knows this viscerally. Can we find the end of practice right here and not project it into the future? A Yoga pose has no end point. Neither does the breath. There are subcurrents in everything, transitional flow, eclipses of eclipses, underwater lava. The "goal of practice" is too utopian and linear a phrase. If we must pour ourselves out completely, we find that what we imagined was a vacuum is actually a fountain. We need this clarifying way of being in the world now more than ever, because we are living in such a human-dominated, human-built world.

At dusk it began raining, and now the evening sky is soft and filled with the dampened sound of a distant airplane. Maybe it's flying hundreds of passengers hundreds of miles home, or away from home, a mile or so above the earth, above cloud, but well beneath the strands of stars that are impossible to make out tonight. Like the sky, the mind is not always clear. We can't sweep away all the clouds of mind, the moods of body, the holding patterns in the nervous system. But we can see them with a mind free of fixation. So waking up is the process of seeing through the cloudiness and the way our attention gets trapped in the clouds of habit. We are always getting caught in these awareness traps. The body is full of them.

If we imagine the earth moving out from between the sun and the moon, and the light returning again to the moon's surface, we have a clear picture of what awakening might mean for us. What is moving out of the way of what? What obscures your ability to remain clear and attentive, present and engaged?

There is an innate stability of awareness and an ongoing feeling of interconnection that comes when we are syncopated with ourselves, syncopated with each other. When we are in time, in rhythm, we are moving with ease, taking action with clarity. Every moment is complete. But not complete in the sense of a final or eternal stillness. The experience of completeness always shifts into something else. Don't get stuck in one state or trait.

We are operating now just as the cloud, as the sand, as the window, as the tree. But of course you are not a tree. You can't ever be a tree. So what does it mean to be human in the same way a tree is being a tree? The tree pulls in light by broadening its canopy while the human stacks wood for the evening fire. When Patañjali says, right in the first paragraph of the *Yoga-Sutra*,

> *Tadā draṣṭu svarūpa vasthānam*
> Then one abides in his or her nature[3]

he is saying that when you can let the distractions that create reactivity just play out without being caught in them, then (*tadā*) you can be yourself, you can abide in your original nature. The term *avasthānam* means "to abide in." But it's not that you are abiding in something you create. It's that the inherent creativity of life moves through you when you are just being yourself.

Living someone else's life is not taking care of your own. Living in another's shadow is to be eclipsed by a life that is not one's own. Sometimes these shadows are our own expectations and judgments. Yoga is about how we live our lives. We must appreciate our finite lives against the backdrop of infinity and interconnectedness. Through our wisdom and long-term practice, we can be anchored in the day-to-day world and find the skillful means necessary for taking care of what we need and also transform our activities into means of service and creative engagement.

Crete, Greece, 2006

11

The Life of a Tulip

Leaning on words
Without a word
A white plum tree's blossomed.
—MUSŌ SOSEKI

IN THE ABOVE verse by Zen poet, calligrapher, monk, and garden designer Musō Soseki (1275–1351), the remarkable, arresting
words make us all come to rest in stillness in this moment. The plum
tree blossoms whether you have words for the process or not. This is
the intelligence of the tree, the mind in life, the life of the mind of
the natural world. This is the great body. Where is this body to be
found? To whom does it belong?

We can't access the great body by looking for it, because it is not
separate from us. Nothing is. The goal of Yoga is to undo the rampant
and unconscious patterns of greed, consumerism, addiction, and in-
attention within and around us by learning how to pay attention, let
go of fixed views, and look after the earth as we care for our own bodies. The heart of our practice is attentiveness and loving action. This
happens within our own bodies and also in everything we do. This is
as much a personal practice as it is a cultural form of awakening.

If religious practices are about inner transformation, and the progressive ecological and social movements are about societal transformation, we need both. Yoga is the waking up of a civilizational matrix. It includes the individual but goes beyond to also take care of our institutions, cities, and plants. Yoga is a practice of human flourishing and community care that leaves the dead end of worldly identification and the fixed views of religion far behind. We do not need commitment to an afterlife or an idea of how the world was created in order to build flourishing cities and take care of one another.

In *āsana* practice we wake up the intelligence of the sense organs through breathing patterns and geometric physical forms in order to clarify our mode of seeing, our mode of being. We don't need practice to realize stillness or interdependence, but we certainly need practice to keep the awareness sustained long enough to transform the habitual drives always moving toward action. We need practice to make our insights real. We need practice to catch the shadows of practice. When we touch the place of stillness that occurs before our world begins, we can gain a kind of clarity that's not possible when we are caught in old patterns of thinking and movement that we have inherited and continue to reinforce. Practice makes life fresh.

Consider these words from an ancient Persian poem:

> These wounds of Cupid, on your heart, Taleba, are not
>   accidental:
> they were engendered by Nature, like the streaks on the
>   leaf of a tulip.[1]

We are all wounded with past karmic patterns engendered by nature, much like the streaks on the leaf of a tulip. This is why karma can be translated as creativity: what are you going to do with what you've inherited? Karma is not something you do—it is something you are. The promise of both Buddhism and Yoga is to wake up to the inherent connection we all have with everything around us. This connection also comes with responsibility, because everything we do has a consequence. The self-focused self is the ultimate cause of *duḥkha* (unsatisfactoriness). The Buddha continually denied the existence of an atomized self separate from the world around us. The heart of the dharma is not being saved by gods or entering heavenly realms but radically transforming the way we experience ourselves and the world around and within us. What is good for me and what is good for others becomes more and more congruent.

If the self *is* karma, it continually changes based on our intentions and choices. The self is steered and created by our attentiveness. This means that at bottom the self is not one thing, be it evil, good, sinful, or joyful. The self has no inherent bottom. What we do becomes what we are. The Buddha describes it this way:

> By action is one a farmer, by action a craftsman,
> By action is one a merchant, by action a servant,
> By action is one a thief, by action a soldier,
> By action is one a priest, by action a ruler,
> In this way the wise see action as it really is,
> Seeing conditioned arising, understanding result of action [2]

The Buddha is not suggesting that karma is something that happens to you or that you are not responsible for your actions. He continues to define the self *as* karma:

> Just as a farmer irrigates his field,
> Just as a fletcher fashions an arrow,
> Just as a carpenter shapes a piece of wood,
> So the sage tames the self.[3]

The Buddha never taught that your karma will create diseases or natural disasters. He calls such an approach to karma "overshooting:"

Moliyasivaka: "Master Gotama, there are some ascetics and brahmins who hold such a doctrine and view as this: 'Whatever a person experiences, whether it be pleasant or painful or neither-painful-nor-pleasant, all that is caused by what was done in the past.' What does Master Gotama say about this?"

"Some feelings, Sivaka, arise here originating from bile disorders: that some feelings arise here originating from bile disorders one can know for oneself, and that is considered to be true in the world. Now when those ascetics and brahmins hold such a doctrine and view as this: 'Whatever a person experiences, whether it be pleasant or painful or neither-painful-nor-pleasant, all that is caused by what was done in the past,' they overshoot what one knows by oneself and they overshoot what is considered to be true in the world. Therefore I say that this is wrong on the part of those ascetics and brahmins."[4]

We are not wounded as the doctrine of original sin suggests. We have in us the potential to wake up as well as the potential to shut down, and we are always alternating between these poles. This is where the form of practice helps. This is also where community helps. Practicing with others helps keep our enthusiasm and energy pointed in the right direction. In this case the right direction has to do with clarifying our relations.

Teachings about turning away from the seductions of the external world are not about distancing from the world of the body and community but rather about getting some perspective on our reactivity. Deeply understanding the conditioned nature of our world allows space for a stance of nonattachment to our reactivity and thus a deeper embrace of the heart of things. "Don't go back over what has passed," the Buddha teaches,

> Nor yearn for what is yet to be.
> What has passed has been abandoned,
> And the future is not yet here.
> The state of arising here and now—
> See it with insight as it is.[5]

In his *Bodhicaryāvatāra* (VIII.26, 28), the poet Śāntideva praises the forest as a delightful place conducive to nonattachment:

Trees do not bear grudges nor is any effort required to please them. When might I dwell with those who dwell happily together? When shall I dwell in the vast regions owned by none, in their natural state, taking my rest or wandering as I please?[6]

The wandering that Śāntideva refers to here helps cultivate the skills necessary to take action in a world out of balance. Nonattachment means engagement. When we wander in the forest, we also have to take care of the forest. If you wander in your neighborhood, you must also take care of it. The intimacy we find in deep practice motivates us to take action. Practice is action. And yet social revolution without inward transformation will not be successful, as we've seen with many revolutions that have replaced one violent regime with another. If we don't look inward and transform our own capacity for greed, violence, and anger, we won't embody the values and vision that we seek to create in the larger social order. On the other side, to view the Yoga and Buddha dharma as a practice divorced from serious social and political change is to miss the primary teachings of those traditions. Just as the self is malleable, so is the culture, the economy, our perspectives on issues. As the Dalai Lama says:

> Destruction of nature and natural resources results from ignorance, greed, and lack of respect for the earth's living things. This lack of respect extends even to the earth's human descendants, the future generations who will inherit a vastly degraded planet if world peace does not become a reality and if destruction of the natural environment continues at the present rate.[7]

In everything we do we are planting seeds. This is creative living. What kind of seeds are you planting? If every action we take is an expression of our practice, each moment is a moment of creative potential. What are you doing with what comes your way? We need a secular dharma. If our personal and collective values are structured, they can be restructured. The term *secular,* derived from the Latin *saecullum*, means "of this time." Can we return to great teachers like Patañjali, Dogen, the Buddha, Śāntideva, Sulak Sivaraksa, Thich Nhat Hanh, Martin Luther King Jr., and others and place them in the social and political realities of their time in order to see them as people responding to the society in which they lived? Reading the lives of these figures in this way allows us to learn about the ways they responded to the conflicts in and around them rather than idealize their cultural surroundings. This gives us a framework for learning how to respond to our times. Today virtually all axial-age civilizations are going through their own distinctive forms of transformation in response to the multiple challenges of modernity. One of the most crucial questions they face is what wisdom they can offer to reorient the developmental trajectory of the modern world in light of the growing environmental crisis.[8] Drawing on the old poets and teachers, we must apply practice to this life at this time. Chinese philosopher Chang Tsai put it this way:

Therefore that which fills the universe I regard as my body and that which directs the universe I consider as my nature. All people are my brothers and sisters, and all things are my companions.[9]

Freedom is the recognition of the intimacy of all things. We don't have to unite any one thing with another, because everything is already whole, already united. For such insight to move into the activities of daily life, we turn to the technique of practice and the support of community and good teachers.

Home, locality, community, and global life are all interconnected with this mind and body sitting here in this room. If the river is polluted, you are polluted. If we have to live in a much larger world, because ecological problems can only be managed on a global scale, the infrastructure between home locality and state is also vital. The infrastructure between body and Earth is most vital. An ecological focus is a necessary corrective to the modernist view that has reduced Yoga and many other spiritual practices to a self-oriented and isolationistic endeavor. Anyone who has gone on retreat knows that in the silence of mind and body, what we tune in to is not some heavenly realm but the vivid realization that all manner of body, speech, and mind interpermeate everything. Culture and the natural world, breath and body, silence and movement, all figure into one another. This is the ecology of Yoga: the streaks of life in the petal of the tulip.

In such a view, everything is sacred. In the appeal of scientists at the Global Forum on Human Development in New York in 1999, religious and spiritual leaders were challenged to envision the human-Earth relationship in a new light:

> As scientists, many of us have had profound experiences of awe and reverence before the universe. We understand that what is regarded as sacred is more likely to be treated with care and respect. Our planetary home should be so regarded. Efforts to safeguard and cherish the environment need to be infused with a vision of the sacred.[10]

While it fully acknowledges that we are embedded in Earth, body, family, and community, Yoga never denies that we are in tune with the cosmic order. To infuse our earthly, bodily, familial, and communal existence with a transcendent significance is not only a lofty ideal but a deep recognition of the continuity of all things. We don't need to make up a cosmic order or metaphysical structure to feel part of this ongoing life force, because when such categories and divisions are dropped, we need only to look around.

Look out the large windows at the little birds lifting high on the breeze over the small grove. This practice may seem difficult at times—stilling your body and mind, paying attention to details, feeling what is really going on in and around us—but the work pays off when the walls of the mind come down and our energy has clarity and stability. When I take care of my anger, my impatience with my son, my tendency to blame others, and my jealousy, I am better able to take action in my family and my life. When I am at ease I am practicing Karma Yoga.

There is no secret language to learn; only this. *Anātman* is not a philosophical position that points to a nonexisting self but rather a map for seeing the world as oneself.

Los Angeles, California, 2004

12

Diversity

Looking after oneself, one looks after others.
Looking after others, one looks after oneself.
—Buddha, Samyutta Nikaya

Although poverty and climate change seem unrelated," writes Paul Hawken in *Blessed Unrest*, "they have common roots for the simple reason that we *are* nature, literally, in every molecule and neuron."[1] In many Yoga postures we viscerally imagine our similarity to nonhuman species. We are living at a time when we need to take care of the world in the same way as we take care of our very own bodies and we need to extend this care to rivers, parents, children, and animals. Nothing should remain outside of our sphere of attentiveness and compassion. After all, selfish happiness is an oxymoron.

In traditional Indian texts like the Upaniṣads and Ṛg Veda, we find the human described in terms of the elements, the elements described in terms of persons and persons redescribed as animals until one finds little distinction between all forms of life. From the *Puruṣa Sūkta:*

The moon was born from his mind;
His eyes gave birth to the sun;

And the wind was born from his breath
From his navel arose the central axis;
From his feet, the earth; from ears, all the directions.
From all of this, the world was formed.[2]

Though similar to a Judeo-Christian creation myth, this passage has a distinct characteristic: namely, the interconnection between the elements of creation in nature and the elements that make up the human being. There is no separation made between Nature's producing organs of perception that make us uniquely human and the creation of the world itself. In his book *Nonviolence to Animals, Earth, and Self in Asian Traditions,* Christopher Chapple follows this theme with a wonderful passage from the *Bṛadāraṇyaka Upaniṣad:*

> As a tree of the forest,
> Just so, surely, is man.
> His hairs are leaves,
> His skin the outer bark.
> From his skin blood,
> Sap from the bark flows forth.
> From him when pierced comes forth,
> A stream, as from the tree when struck.
> His pieces of flesh are under-layers of wood.
> The fiber is muscle-like, strong.
> The bones are wood within.
> The marrow is made resembling pith.[3]

In this poem, "his hairs are leaves" is not a metaphor. It is not a comparison. The leaves do not stand for anything. When we look at a river it *is* the body, not a sign for some other thing.

Our religions have devised innumerable and imaginative ways to explain the creation of the world and our purpose here in this lifetime. The truth of such connections opens us up to an ancient mystery. The English word *nature* is derived from the Latin *natura,* meaning "birth" or "constitution." It is further derived from the term *nat,* which is where we get the words *native, nation, and natal.*

The important denominator in these aspects of the word *nature* is that it means *everything.* The natural wilderness and function of one's own mind and body are not etymologically distinct from the great fir forests or the ocean currents or the current of breath streaming through the nostrils as you read these words.

Paul Hawken continues his description of the inseparability of the designations *human* and *nature:*

> We contain clay, minerals, and water, are powered by sunshine through plant life; and are intricately bound to all other species, from fungi to marsupials to bacteria. In our lungs are oxygen molecules breathed by every type of creature ever to have lived on earth, along with the very hydrogen and oxygen atoms that Jesus, Confucius, and Rachel Carson breathed.[4]

Being part of a vast ecosystem brings moral responsibility. If our spiritual practice does not respond to the questions posed by the precise forms of *duḥkha* in this time, our practice is misguided. If we are truly seeing a contemporary Yoga develop, it must be alive and adaptable in the current world. Yoga involves a constant opening toward the places where there is suffering—be it in mind, body, culture, or other parts of the ecosystem. Furthermore, practice means feeling an obligation to respond to such suffering even if there is some risk or uncertainty about the outcome of our actions. And although the *yamas*—nonharming, honesty, nonstealing, wise use of energy, and nongreed—offer us a framework for tuning in to the effects of our actions in the matrix of life, they do not provide specific answers to specific situations. The answers are our personal response. How we respond to a situation is contextual and must be appropriate. Giving attention to what's actually going on is really a process of creative engagement. It's not a top-down ethical approach based on vows, precepts, or rules. Giving attention to something is to open ourselves creatively. Meditation in action—in the form of attentiveness and suspending our preconceptions—becomes a situational ethics. What to do cannot be determined by some overarching law. Although sometimes we would like the ethics of practice to be fundamental precepts or absolute commandments, the *yamas* do not offer us any final say in a given matter. Instead they orient us toward a personal response in a given context.

Context is crucial in ethical decisions. A decision has to take into account the background and the conditions that give rise to it. The *yamas* are guidelines for wisdom and compassion, leading the practitioner over and over again into the reality of union and the commitment to taking action. But the *yamas* do not do the work for us. Ultimately we must let the framework fall away in order to open to a practice of true situational ethics.

When practitioners undertake the practice of Yoga and mature through various limbs of practice, ethics, meditation, postures, and breathing techniques, the limbs begin to support one another. Our approach to practice should be taken seriously, and we must always ensure that what we are practicing or teaching as a path is both relevant in contemporary times and will lead to the liberation promised by tradition. Tradition, like ethics, is not "pure"—it is always retouched and revisioned through cultural contact. There is no one pure Yoga system that has survived without alteration. Systems are contingent on the culture in which they are created and practiced. It is crucial for our traditions of Yoga that we can engage with them personally and culturally and remain open to the possibility of Yoga's changing us. We must also wrestle with tradition in order to make it come alive in the here and now.

Nature always comes alive, because it leaves nothing out. Our Yoga should be practiced this way also. The human capacity for compartmentalization is profoundly disturbing. We need a well-rounded practice of ethics, self-care, attention to body and breath, and meditation so that all aspects of our lives are touched by practice. The physical postures alone cannot solve our diverse forms of craving and conflict. When we practice with attention to all the limbs of Yoga, we can bring wisdom to our relationships both internally and externally. Patañjali offers tools for various areas of our lives, not just one technique. "Then," Patañjali declares, "one is no longer disturbed by the play of opposites."[5]

When I go to workshops in Europe or elsewhere, I always look around the room and consider the age range and the feel of the group. Usually there is diversity. While I think it's important to engage with the rigors of intellectual debate with contemporary forms of philosophy and science, the practices of Yoga have to work at a visceral level as well. I don't always know which side to land on: expansive and flexible, or traditional and fixed. At different times both styles of practice are needed. To return us to the subject of Yoga, ethics and the natural world, the classical texts and practices need to come alive in our life. This is the essential point. If our practice is not bringing us into active engagement with our life, it's missing the target. With incense and chanting or without, we all have to figure out how to bring our commitment to practice into everyday life in a way that serves. This is the heart of intimate practice.

For Yoga to be light on its feet, it has to speak to people without technical jargon and elitism. I have made this statement before, and I don't know if it's true. I struggle with a contradiction in my presentation of Yoga and also in myself. Sometimes I know it's there, and sometimes I can't see it at all. Why do I write: "it has to speak to people without technical jargon and elitism" and then go on to use terms like *situational ethics* and *existential disorientation*. A friend was at another public talk I gave, and someone turned to her at the end and described how he was going through a divorce and the teachings were really helping him and he wanted to share with me what he was learning. But he felt intimidated because he couldn't talk to me in a way that "was smart enough." Sometimes I am teaching simple Yoga dharma, sometimes we are dropping our thighs in forward bends, and sometimes I am immersed in the nuances of postmodern cultural studies. As much as I try to practice in a very simple way, I can't undo the way I understand myself and the language that I use. Cultural theory and art-school rhetoric actually speak to my experience of myself more than any other language. I am constantly reading poetry and academic books.

When I teach I am always shifting back and forth between silent practice and rigorous dialogue and thinking. I want to teach simple postures and meditations in which little or no language is needed, and then I also want to explore what this means for my own life, and possibly yours, and in order to do so I need to speak in a language in which I am comfortable. I am comfortable in going back and forth between academic talk and self-help. I need both in my own life. Maybe that's why I talk like this.

Many musicians say that the depth of meaning in music is too precise for words. Meditation teachers say the same thing about silence. Of course I agree, but at the same time, I live in a sea of language I cannot escape, and so when I use words, I want to use them with accuracy. I don't want to say the snow is cold and white. I want to enter the snow and then come back with words that communicate clearly. So I write a lot about snow. Right now Vienna is free of snow. But last week at the airport in Frankfurt, there was no wind and the snow looked like feathers falling slowly to earth, as if a pillow fight were happening straight above me. I mention this because sometimes I get very self-conscious about pressing myself to use language in new ways. Perhaps you could say this is a writing prompt or a technique, but for me, it reaches further beyond that—it's a way to move deep into the world. This helps me to see with clearer eyes, revealing the undisguised vastness of this moment.

When a woman sat beside me on the plane from Germany and asked me what I did, I was embarrassed to say "Yoga teacher." I don't see myself wearing leotards on the cover of a Yoga DVD at the check-out line at Whole Foods. Sometimes I want to reach everyone buying those DVDs and at other times I want to participate in the political and intellectual movements that can change the paradigms of society. I want to be truthful in unwinding my experience so that others can see their own lives in new ways. This requires a constantly shifting vocabulary.

When a snowflake drops onto my outstretched palm, its body disintegrates immediately. Tiny rivulets flow from its melting form. This morning, I can see snowflakes on the sidewalk for only a split second. When stillness arises, movement shows up immediately.

Vienna, Austria, 2007

13

Waves and Water:
Form and Freedom

You (Bodhisattva) and Wisdom (prajñā) are essentially
the same,
Like pearls rolling on a tray, light, random, uninhibited.
—HAKUIN ZENJI, COMMENTARY ON THE
HEART-SUTRA

SPONTANEITY IS THE functional movement of clear seeing. Spontaneity is the wild and untaught dharma, the free and un-hindered expression of Yoga. And as you hear these words, the fish are swimming it, the musicians are playing it, the poets are putting it down on napkins. Our culture has taught us how to be effective, how to work, and how to keep busy. But perhaps there is a way to be active in our lives without the burnout and stress that characterize active lives. Maybe we need to learn how to let things be without becoming passive. Doesn't that sound like a paradox?

Cultivating attention might be a new way of creating stability in our lives and relationships. Attentiveness is also an important fea-ture of a creative life.

In the story "Hikai no Go," in the *Yamato Monogatari,* the pro-tagonist announces that a poem will be composed that requires a final hemstitch and asks that the great artists all come out to hear the poem and then respond with a capping verse. Here is the first part of the poem:

> Why is the small deer
> standing right in the middle
> of the open sea?

To which a student who was in attendance added:

> I think the autumn mountains
> are clearly reflected there.[1]

An outrageously clear response. Look closely at those mountains in autumn and there you'll see the deer, grazing in the sea.

"Like beads rolling on a tray," Hakuin writes in his commentary on the *Heart Sūtra*, "light, random, uninhibited."[2] Please move beyond the outer form of the Yoga postures, the perfection of body image, the sequential and mechanical movement of learned poses, so you can see what they are pointing at. John should not practice like Ali, and David should not practice like Basia. Creative expression is as boundless as freshly cut grass—all of those green blades ready to sprout: always ready, always sprouting.

Right now life manifests as the small ant crawling upward along the bookshelf, the river trout returning from the lake back to the waters not far from this very building, the heron circling above the Chinese restaurant where we all ate today. Spatially and temporally you can be in every one of those bodies—we all exist equally and simultaneously. You can imagine yourself right now as the tractor operator outside and also as a politician walking the cabinet floor in the parliament buildings down the road. It's helpful to stop what we are engaged in once in a while and imagine ourselves as the paint on the wall or the infant crawling along in a sandbox somewhere. This is life operating, pushing forward, moving time. You *are* time. No separation.

DEATH AND THE SINGULAR SELF

I've been asked to address concerns about dying in relation to the flow of life. There is the feeling of "I" as the one who dies; the singular "me" is no longer going to be participating in the forward momentum of life. My feeling in response to that is, well, who is dying? The singular moves back into the plural, the infinite. From one perspective, the singular returns to the infinite at death. But the singular is dying every moment. The singular is never one thing. Change is a continuous seamless web, and moments come, maybe even this one, when you feel stuck in one particular way, or as one exact thing. If we can understand that dying and change are happening moment to moment, then death is not projected into the future. We tend to think that death is going to happen to me in the future. But death is replacing life in each moment. And also, let's not forget that the singular was never separate to begin with. So on the one hand we can't deny the singular nature of a human life. And on the other hand, we need to see that singularity against the backdrop of a conditioned world in flux, where everything is interconnected with everything else back through beginningless time and forward for as far as we can imagine. Freud says we repress death.[3] But from a yogic perspective what we repress is not a death projected into the future but the fact that the singular self never existed in the first place. Like a wave, it is a momentary phenomenon empty of substantiality. You were never here to begin with! We are relational, ecological, biological contingencies. The self is added afterward. Again, the singular self is not just something that dies in the future but also, truly, something that never really had a separate life of its own in the first place.

COMMUNITY AND THE INDIVIDUAL SELF

Traditional Indian texts divide the witness from what is observed, much like the way we can divide the subject from the object or spirit from matter. The seer and the seen are like waves and water—they are varied forms of the same flow. Flow is transient and also eternal—going on and on, on and on. One of the tools we employ at Centre of Gravity is to work in pairs, asking one another questions and engaging in active listening. After some quiet periods of meditation practice, we break into pairs, sit facing each other, and ask each other simple and direct questions like "Who are you?" "What hindrances are arising for you?" "What stops you?"

This is a very intimate practice. And it's hard because of the way it shows us where we hold on, where we're fixed, where we are too self-conscious. It's taken many years for me to relax during these exercises and learn to share with others the interior working of my own life. This form of expression is challenging because it becomes very obvious when we are not speaking honestly, when our social persona is dominant. When resistance arises, the flow of the dialogue breaks down and sometimes stops altogether. Part of this practice is to express ourselves honestly and spontaneously, "like beads rolling on a tray: light, random, and uninhibited." This is a combination of *satya* (honesty) and *svādhyāya* (self-study). We study our patterns so we can forget about them.

One of the reasons we engage in this group process is obvious: so we can each recognize and articulate what we may be caught up in during our practice periods and our lives. On another level, we are also learning how to practice true self-expression—how to express ourselves in an unhurried, unrehearsed, and spontaneous, heartfelt way.

It's too easy to practice in an interior personalized world in which we are not pushed to express our realization in language with others. We are always humans, and so our experience is shared through language. Practice divorced from this sharing leaves out the interrelational aspect of life. It's easy to remain interior with our contemplative practices, but it's challenging to communicate our experience, listen to others, and learn how to activate our practice in communication with others. And I'm not just talking about speaking with a friend about your Yoga postures—I mean sharing what arises for you on the mat, on the cushion, in everyday relations. Friendship is the heart of this way of practicing. It's necessary to challenge ourselves to practice in this way so that our lives are integrated, so parts of the body speak with one another, so the cast of inner characters and compulsions can tend to one another. We practice in this way to bring compartmentalization to an end.

We are living wisdom in everything we say and do. A compassionate action is not done with wisdom, it *is* wisdom. You are not cultivating compassion—you *are* compassion. Wisdom and compassion are essentially the same. When we are uninhibited, we express our basic nature, and this comes alive in a community of fellow practitioners and beings. Freedom is illusory if it's not lived, not acted upon, not felt continuously in our interpersonal interactions. This is your life. This is my life. This is life. This is community. You *are* community. *Sangha* is ciphered through all the intricate dependencies of our lives.

The world is vast and the body and breath are spacious when we are at ease with others and ourselves. This ease comes through committed practice, in which we learn how to open to the life of the body, the situations of others, and the moods that move through us with equanimity and creativity. Don't get stuck. Don't go ahead. Just stop and look at the type on this page, the quality of light in the room where you are, the sounds in the distance. This is where you enter. Each sound is a pearl, a treasure, a wave that brings you back to your body. There is nothing subtle to find. Look at the walls and the crack in the ceiling. Look at all the cracks and the fine woodwork and the realness of the real that pervades all we are doing. All of this is a gift. Set forth this miraculous gift. How do you set it forth? How do you express Yoga? In what you do. In the way you see and hear and breathe. This is the true expression of our practice. This is how we activate our practice.

THE INTERRELATIONAL SELF

Self-reflection must take us beyond the self. Self-reflection (*svādhyāya*) moves us deep into the world. In ancient times the philosophy of subjective study was called *ānvīkṣikī*, which means "what to look at." This refers to what we keep in view. If we are not fragmenting what we see according to personal preferential criteria, we can keep more of our lives in view.

Keeping everything in view includes the sphere of speech. When we don't feel secure with a loved one, usually we either ramp up our attempts to get a reaction from the person or we dismiss our own needs in an attempt to become impervious to what's happening.

A friend who has studied Yoga for many years was becoming increasingly unhappy in her marriage because her partner had very little sexual energy for her, and so she continually imagined that her desire was bad. She had to overcome her sexual needs. In fact, the more she studied at a monastery she was visiting in the summers, the more she was supported in this view by the notion that sexual desire is "unwholesome." Although she and I talked at length about the way sexual desire was not the problem and the real cause of suffering was clinging and craving, this did not help. What was distressing to her was that she most feared expressing to her husband that she desired him, that her needs were going unmet, that she wanted to be with him and didn't know how anymore. She was scared to drop into how she felt and express it honestly.

Not speaking honestly is a form of disengagement, not genuine Yoga. When we look clearly, we are able to find our friend or lover behind the narrow image we've created for the person. Sometimes he or she may not even know what we're feeling or needing. When withdrawers can move toward a more open and vulnerable stance and when blamers can ask for their needs to be met in a sincere way, we can begin to include more of one another in our shared speech.

This relational way of thinking about attention is re-visioning classical Yoga in the light of current thinking about the way our "selves" are relational and linguistic. Language and communication through their patterns are the media in which we live. Patañjali wrote nothing specific on relational language. And yet we have a framework in classical Yoga for breaking through patterns of enmeshment or codependency by becoming more flexible in our responses, by becoming better regulators of our emotions and anxieties, stronger and more confident in ourselves. Bringing Yoga into our personal lives creates a powerful arena for change. I'd like to say this is an act that occurs spontaneously, but I think it's worth emphasizing that meditation is not just turning inward on our cushions. Like many meditators, my tendency when there is trouble in my relationships is to sit still and follow my breath. But that's not always what's needed. Another aspect of the practice is to link the equanimity we cultivate in meditation to our communications with others. Attention training, which is the heart of meditation practice, can be used to tune in to one another while also creating a secure base in ourselves, because we are grounded and less hostile or reactive. Though I learned so much from studying with Asian and Indian teachers, I've needed to embrace the insights of Western psychology in order to tend to the way patterns of habit show up in my relationships.

Along with the biological and internal components of suffering, suffering has interpersonal components: separation from people you love, being with people who agitate you, unresolved conflicts, and unrequited needs. Interpersonal suffering is an important aspect of all suffering. The hungers for pleasure in relationships, to be seen or admired by others, or to hide or escape—these are all causes of suffering. The causes of discontent can be fueled by not seeing our feelings and needs as they really are. When we can't see others, they suffer also. When we look around, we want our lives to be in focus; when we look up at night, we want to see more than just a few dull stars. Sometimes we don't want to look at the interpersonal nature of our entanglements because it's complex, it involves honest self-reflection and also communication with the other. True nonviolence happens right at the precipice of conflict, when we are forced to communicate honestly what is really going on within and around us, both with ourselves and with others.

The key factor in all relationships, whether in relation to our economy, to our lover, or even to ourself, is how moments of disconnection are handled. When we can still our reactivity, we can see the logic behind our choices, and we also have space enough in our hearts and minds to tolerate disconnection, aloneness, anger, or abandonment. This tolerance is essential for relational attunement.

Yoga teaches us how to open to difference so that conflict does not define our relationships.

The movement of the waves, the movement of the body—this is the truth of transience. This life is precious, as is every dawn, every breath. It's an incredible gift to be able to live your life with this awareness. That's why we practice—not to be reminded of temporary feelings of intimacy but to see that we live as the water and function as the wave. What is your life about? This wisdom connects us back with our heart.

The inhalation waves through you and the exhale washes over the pelvic floor, then leaves the body. You are born, you become a wave, and then you recede. But you are never separate from water. Waves have the quality of water in every movement. Waves and water cannot be separated. You are a wave and life is water. You may have unique characteristics, but you are not an independent entity. Everything that exists is whispered through our breath, courses through our bloodstream, and adheres to our changing cells.

In death there is this same kind of shift. One thing ceases and another thing starts. Of course we are not functioning anymore as the wave in the water. We become the water completely. We move back into the elements. In death we give completely, until we are not functioning relative to the whole; we *are* the whole.

Lessons in death and dying can influence how we conduct our daily life here, moment-to-moment, activity-to-activity, and person-to-person. In light of death, how can you and I speak honestly? Ikkyu, the famous Zen master, went to see one of his lay friends who was dying. He told him: "I will now guide you to your last end." The man, a Zen disciple, said: "I don't need your guidance. I came alone, I go alone." Ikkyu said: " If you think you came alone and you go alone, that's your illusion. I'll teach you where there is no coming and no going." And the man, when he heard that, smiled and died.[4]

Coming and going, like life and death, are irrelevant phrases when we are fully in our lives. The sunset does not die, it becomes a sunrise somewhere else. Here in Washington State, where I am writing, the glaciers to the north are flowing by in mad white water. The water climbing up the banks reminds me that when we die, we just die. Nothing added. There is a story about Tozan, when he was dying.[5] A monk asked him: "Master, is there somebody who is not sick?" He said, "Yes, there is somebody who is not sick." The monk: "Does this person, who is not sick, look at you?" And the master said, "It is not for him to look at me, it is for this old monk to look at him." The monk asked, "How do you look at him, at him who is not sick?" The master: "When I look at him who is never sick, there is no sickness at all." So that is a way of saying, there is also somebody in me who is never sick, who is beyond sickness and dying. But this is very abstract and philosophical, even for the meditator who can face pain. Tokusan, another Zen master, was asked the same question on his deathbed: "Is there somebody who is not sick?" He said: "Yes, there is." And then the monk asked: "How do you look at him?" And Tokusan said, *"Aaooah, aaooah aah."* He was in distress. There is really no difference between the one who is not sick and the one who is. This is the core of Yoga and is what is meant by the terms *yoke* or *intimacy* or *samādhi*. Waves and water, body and mind.

ETHICAL RESPONSIVENESS

Flexibility and spontaneity are terms we talk about a lot. But can we really shift in all of our life situations so that we can meet each moment as it happens? Nothing stays the same. Even what we think of as "me" and "mine" is a shifting variation. I can't be the same Michael I am in this room while teaching as when I'm at home with my son trying to tape a cardboard door onto the fort he's made behind our couch. You can't be the same person in *prāṇāyāma* that you are when you are changing diapers. You shouldn't be. What's important about this practice is letting go, so you can let this practice shift to meet each situation as it presents itself. This movement is flow, the flow of all life. Conditions change; so must you. I call this situational ethics:

the ability to respond to what's right in front you. If we can begin to see that ethical responsiveness has everything to do with our attentiveness and our ability to let go of fixed views, we can start to see how ethics (*yamas*) are an expression of *samādhi* (interconnectedness, integration). We depend on letting go in order to remember what we need to know.

In the same way that there is no fixed self, there are also no fixed laws of activity that guarantee peaceful outcomes. There are no ethics in general; there are only fluid processes through which we enter a situation. Turning down our reactivity allows us to enter situations more fully. Ethics show up every day in every decision. This is one of the reasons why being able to see through the distractions (*citta-vṛtti*) of consciousness and stay steady in body and heart becomes a moral discipline, a responsibility to others.

As we've explored in detail, what constitutes our image of ourselves is a subjective story that we construct over the course of our lives, and others help us create it as well. A subject only remains a subject because the person constantly rearticulates himself or herself. We can all feel what it's like to rehash old stories of ourselves and others that are stale. And yet we continue to do so through a kind of addiction to gluing and lacquering old stories, as we paste ourselves together moment to moment, like some kind of collage. Societies and nations do this as well, through creating identity and enemies. After a time, it becomes hard to shift the groove of these stories. The coherence of a story depends on repetition. What is so powerful about attentiveness as a practice is that it disrupts these habitual stories so we can enter our lives more fully. According to both the Yoga and the Buddhist traditions, many of these stories are rooted in fear, which is itself rooted in the three poisons: greed, anger, and confusion.

There's so much anger, desire and self-judgment, greed, shame, and momentum in each of our lives—both individually and as a whole. Yoga is learning how to take care of these energies, to find proximity with them rather than identify with them. We can create momentum in new directions so that spaciousness arises. Momentum and countermomentum give way to transformation.

The psychology of this process is to see the way greed, anger, and delusion create the momentum of suffering (*duḥkha*) in our lives and communities. Yoga and Buddhism distinguish between wholesome and unwholesome (*kusala* and *akusala*) tendencies and identify the primary sources of unwholesome behavior as greed, anger, and delusion. It is not difficult to see how these three work together: my greed reinforces my anger toward those who obstruct it, and both reinforce my sense of separation from others; my delusion of separation also reinforces my greed and thus my anger. Their interaction creates the *duḍkha* of bad karma, affecting not only me but those around me. To really transform *duḥkha*, greed, anger, and delusion need to be transformed into their positive counterparts: greed into generosity, ill will into loving-kindness, delusion into wisdom.

NAMES AND FORMS

The mind is constantly caught up in the identity of name (*nāma*) and form (*rūpa*). This is good. The initial differentiation that comes through naming things is very helpful. Name has to do with our conditioning of each and every moment. Name doesn't just constitute something in language but has to do with our feelings about things, the meaning we give things, the way we focus on a particular task. So how we name things has more to do with idiom or character.[6] The *rūpa* in *nāma-rūpa* refers to organic matter (the matter that enters into the composition of the living being). So *rūpa* is a material form that refers to the four primary elements of matter: earth or solidity, fire or heat, water or cohesion, air or movement.

So when we sit, we can experience the moment-to-moment impermanent nature of all the elements. We have the heat, the air, the water, the thoughts, and feelings. So what elements can you truly consider to be your own body if you truly look at it just as elements arising and passing away on a moment-to-moment level? Try to grasp hold of any one of those elements, try to hang on to one, even just one sensation in the body, and say "That is me." It is impermanent. When we contemplate the body, we can experience that microscopic level of that constant change and flux, bubbles, atoms. And we can experience this directly. There is no permanent, separate entity called "self" there in all those elements. And that constant changing, that state of flux, is what we mean by waves and water being mutually dependent.

Underneath the names we give forms, the natural world moves forward in its own patterning. The rivers are in compliance with the spring—we heard them rushing last night. The snow has melted, and now the birds are spreading their little voices everywhere. The baby-leaf soft breath of that little bird is also your own breath. It's the wind in everything. Your fleshy belly, the diving gulls, the relentless tractors outside—this is one great body operating infinitely. What you do anywhere in the body affects every other part. There's no telling where your breath ends and mine begins, where the blood in your spleen ends and the maple syrup begins. Dragonflies have butterfly wings. Tear ducts look like sewage ducts.

Where is the nose? Where is the body? Where is the self? Of course we can tag the location of these "things," but when we look into the body with our eyes closed, we slice the awareness thinner and thinner until we see that sensations do not arise in the body at all. They arise in awareness. There is no thing that *is* body. Body is a shifting flow in time and space. This frees us. We can get so locked into thinking that there is something called Michael in his body, Sharon in her body, Simone in her body. But what are all of these bodies? Grasping and rejecting both give rise to suffering. We can understand that. There is a way out of this contraction, but this is not something to believe. Rather than believing Patañjali, we employ his technique, we embody the teachings, so that we can see.

So much of our self-generated human suffering is believing the language that we use. Sadly, I have bulldozed through so many relationships because I have been firm in my analysis of the other person—my analysis a form of blame. I believed in my viewpoint so strongly. I held on to my ideas—and I still do sometimes—in ways that shut down listening. No intimacy is possible when we are accusatory or fixed in our view.

Over time we begin to see that language, like rivers or veins, can get clogged up. And since Yoga is practiced in three realms—body, speech, and mind—we are continually unclogging these routes of human perception and expression. The obstacles that we meet—in the form of self-judgment, inadequacy, or whatever your unique obstacles are—are not separate from reality. *Samsāra* is nirvana, *avidyā* is *vidyā* (seeing clearly). The *koti* (limit, boundary) of nirvana is the *koti* of *samsāra*. Awakening and delusion are mutually dependent. What shuts us down (*samsāra*) is actually the very path that opens us up (nirvana). They are two different ways of experiencing this world. Nirvana is not another realm or dimension but rather the clarity and peace that arise when our mental turmoil ends, because the objects with which we have been identifying are realized to be *Śūnya* (boundless). Things have no reality of their own that we can cling to, since they arise and pass away according to conditions. Nor can we cling to this truth. Vaśiṣṭha describes this to the confused sage Rama:

> The distinction between ripples and the water is unreal and verbal. Even so, the distinction between ignorance and knowledge is unreal and verbal. There is neither ignorance here nor even knowledge! When you cease to see knowledge and ignorance as two distinct identities, what exists, alone exists.[7]

Of course the language we use to describe "things" is not the thing in itself. But at the same time, language itself is sacred.

When I was caught in anger regarding a story about my father in one retreat, I had a meeting with the teacher, who told me sternly: "Thoughts about your father are NOT your father." This was so freeing. I kept telling myself stories about my father that kept erupting into anger, and she was telling me to stop focusing on the projected and learn about the projector instead. This is a very hard thing to do. I think that what I think is fact. But when I let down the fortress walls in mind and body, I can see the way life really happens. My father appears as he is. My quarrels with him don't come to an end, but my reactivity does. I love him in his faults.

You are not what your parents think you are. You are not what your teacher thinks you are. But who are you? How do you express who you are? There is a comfort in "knowing who and what we are," but this obstructs the freedom of moment-to-moment flow. Deep in the wisdom of free seeing is interconnectedness. But we express this interconnectedness through action and language. Otherwise insight coagulates, as does anything that is not expressed. Meiko Matsudaira writes:

> Passion unspoken
> congeals,
> growing into a black pearl
> deep
> in my body.[8]

Our Yoga practice wakes these pearls up from slumber in body, speech, and mind. Taking care of ourselves, we take care of one another. There are a million ways to take care of the world, a million ways to serve. But we need to be *here* for this expression. I am hungry and getting my coat off the back of this chair as I prepare to go out for another meal, and as I do so, I observe this body right here, this breath, the food and garden along this wonderful road. As I walk and talk with Susan, we ask ourselves: Where does seeing take place? Where is seeing? Who is seeing?

There is no substantiality in any one thing. You do not have a nature separate from any river or any material conditions. When we shift our patterns of perception, we shift our patterns of behavior. This shift in seeing helps us get unstuck. Nothing has a solid sense, everything is temporary, and all life is interrelational. All aspects and elements of life have these qualities. We are all attenuated and massaged not just by free independent will but through the cocreation of everything and everyone. This is vast interconnectedness. Like a pearl rolling on a tray, our job is to keep up with how we feel and express ourselves when the time is right: sudden, ready, uninhibited.

The highest goal of modern Yoga is to point out how there is a natural intimacy embedded within everything no matter how large or small, and when we forget this intimacy of which we are a part, we have practices to remind us again and again that everything we do makes a difference. While modern technology like airplanes, indoor climate control, and iPhones actually place the individual outside the natural cycles and responsibilities of life, coming back to our bodies and cultivating attentiveness can work to undo those stratifications within and around the human-built world. Humanity is like the flora and fauna of the natural world, and we need to slow down and pay attention so that we don't continually forget the responsibilities that come from being part of such a vast community. Nobody can simply act on his or her own behalf. The world is too deeply interconnected for any of us to continue full speed ahead with only egoic desires in mind. I find great comfort in knowing that we are never alone.

The middle path in Yoga is the *suṣumnā*—the great central axis that connects heaven and breath, breath and mind, beginning and end, life and death. In terms of the body, this central axis is the path in that this is where we follow the movements of breath and mind so that our surface distractions can settle within the body. The body is just the body. The world dangles in front of your eyelashes—just have a look. When you leave here, please rush into the world. Can you break through the body into the body? Can you break through your marriage and go into marriage? Study your body until you grasp it. And when you grasp it, let it go again. You can't hold on to the path.

Ottawa, Canada, 2008

PART THREE

Formal Practice

14

Encouragement on Retreat

The universe and I exist together, and all things and I
are one. Since all things are one what room is there for
speech? But since I have already said that all things are
one, how can speech not exist?
—CHUANG-TZU, "SEEING THINGS AS EQUAL"

WE ARE NOT LIVING in times that require more ideology
or philosophy. And yet I feel compelled to speak philosophi-
cally. Why? Ideas help shape the way I perceive my life. Practice helps
me let go of those ideas. Practice cannot be divorced from our ideas
of practice, and so we need to continually learn about what practice
is and how it works in our lives.

One of the most compelling aspects of this concentric path of
Yoga is that we can enter the intimacy of reality each and every moment only when we are free of congealed ideas. Although we usually
conceive of "attachment" or "clinging" in terms of objects (money,
home, lovers, friends), Yoga teachings remind us that what we are
most reluctant to give up is not material objects but rather our cher-
ished viewpoints. Across the road from my house is a run-down
home I call the Sorauren Street Drug House. The father is a dealer, he
yells at his two overweight kids all day, and the mother walks the

drugs to the corner when someone calls. I want to call the police. I worry that one day there will be a gunfight in my front yard. But I also see that calling the police may be the worst thing for the kids. I think about it every morning when they're being yelled at on their way down the front stairs, the father's voice pushing them from behind. Though I want him to stop dealing, I worry that without his income the family would sink into a much worse state. It's hard deciding to do nothing. The eaves trough is falling off the side of the roof and the storm windows are all cracked. The small bike on the porch with red training wheels is rusting and never used. I want the best for this family, especially the young kids.

It's our viewpoint that is held to with tremendous energy, and it's clinging to a view that most obscures the inherent intimacy that we all long for. When I don't think about calling the cops and I just stay with all of my feelings, I feel very connected with those kids. I find myself saying hi to them more often.

Intimacy, or love, is not dependent on feeling a certain way. We can love someone and simultaneously not want to be near him or her. The term *Yoga* may be derived from the root *yuj* (to unite), but once it's out of its verb form, it refers to the inherent intimacy of all things. There is nothing we have to actually unite. Every "thing" already interpermeates every other "thing." There is, in fact, no such thing as a thing.

Almost 80 percent of our food supply depends on the life-giving routine of pollinators like the common honeybee. Even the dairy industry, which we imagine to be far from the world of the beehive, is totally dependent on plants that are pollinated by the bees. Likewise, the human immune system is an extraordinarily complex system that relies on an elaborate and dynamic communications network that exists among the many different kinds of immune system cells that patrol the body. This communications network within the body of plants, animals, and humans reminds us of the vast matrix we find ourselves living in.

Perhaps "living in" doesn't accurately describe what and who we are. We *are* this natural communications network in every layer and warp of our lives—there is no way to separate ourselves from the blueberries, pumpkins, winds, and water that sustain our every movement. This interpermeation is Yoga. Yoga is the nonseparation of life: breath and body, body and mind, word and deed, action and stillness.

Our theories about Yoga can't ever capture the vastness of life. Our exploration of Yoga theory, method, and practice always oscillates between technical detail and the vast mystery of life that spreads out when we know when to drop technique and be with life as it really is.

When we sit down together after long days of silent practice, sitting meditation, *prāṇāyāma,* and *āsana,* it's interesting to watch how our energy is very stable, attentive, and enthusiastic. We struggle sometimes during these days of retreat practice: we alternate between the natural stillness that occurs in quietude and the turbulent thoughts that precede this softness. This struggle is our practice. I don't mean that practice is a struggle, but that as the pendulum swings between stillness and distraction, we untie an important knot. Don't underestimate the power of pure awareness. Just by acknowledging the presence of defensiveness, or joy, we invite it more fully into awareness. From there, the knots begin undoing by themselves. This kind of bare and simple recognition of what is cuts through our reactive struggles and escape mechanisms. We can be fully awake in the midst of anything. Like waves in the ocean, even our strongest thought patterns arise and fade away into the vast interconnectedness that composes everything. The waves subside back into the ocean, the cloud back into the sky.

The knot (*granthi*) refers to the habitual reactive patterns in mind and body that occur when we entangle ourselves in too much mental elaboration. When we come together like this to reflect on practice, we do so in order to return to our basic motivation for practice in the first place. This is, of course, different for each of us. It's too simplistic to say we practice to be free or we practice to find our true nature. What's more interesting is to find the unique and personal question that brought *you* to this practice in the first place. The danger of not maintaining contact with our initial questions is that we can lose touch with our intention to practice. And intention is an extremely clarifying element of alignment.

When I was twenty I was pulled under by depression. I left university and then eventually left my job. Life and work and school promised security, but I felt that what I most needed was an absence of human interaction and expectation. I found a silence that was uncomfortable and anxious. What interested me was why silence was so uncomfortable and anxious. I made a vow to learn how to be still, and I decided early one March to steal away, alone, and not to return until I could be still.

I moved to Algonquin Park and lived out of a VW van. Because it was so cold, I actually lived in the van. I clearly remember my first night there, watching the sun die in the clear sky and wondering if I'd be able to stay warm through the night. I was broke, depressed, and lost. I had left my job and my apartment in Birmingham, Michigan. Every morning I woke up cold and lonely. But I was also comforted by the sound of thawing and splitting ice on the frozen lakes thundering me awake each morning. I had no friends in those lost hills and forests, but I was comforted by my resolution to read and sit and practice Yoga. I was going to find peace without conditions.

One morning the battery in the van died and I couldn't warm up. I was so angry that I walked down to a tree and kicked it and realized my toes were still asleep and my legs were freezing. In my rage, I couldn't even feel my body. Then the lake ice cracked. The silent forests echoed that splitting sound over and over. In that moment it occurred to me that the van could be fixed easily but that my toes, the tree, my emotion, my body, were all innocent. I realized that things could happen in my life that I could deal with—like the battery's dying—but that there were also aspects of my experience that I didn't have the skill to be with, to transform, to meet vividly.

That's when I committed myself to practice. When I saw that I could be overwhelmed by life, I also saw that what was overwhelming was not the *circumstance* but what I did with the circumstance. I spent the next week sitting still and really struggling to try to open to the sounds of the lake without too much distraction. This was the beginning of my sitting practice.

Sometimes, after a day like this, I get self-conscious about telling these personal stories, and once in a while I vow never to share them again. But then I remember interviewing a famous teacher at his home and discussing his anxieties and the vexing feelings that prevented him from sitting for years. When the interview was over, he wanted me to erase the parts of our long conversation where he shared his anxieties. He didn't want me to share in public his difficulties meditating. Yet what I heard in his story was the very human difficulty that motivates our practice in the first place. In fact, his honesty inspired me.

We are in a wonderful rural setting, and right now it's interesting to notice how many days it takes to settle into the environment without walking around in a daze. But eventually, when stillness comes, each tree, each sound, each cloud, each voice, can be traced back to its source. And what is the source? If we let go of our ideas about divinity or creation, we can appreciate the interconnection of all these ingredients. And the ingredients include each and every one of us. You are uniquely you, but you are also a corner of the universe that we call flow, that we call life.

We often chant this line at the start of our day:

Yoga citta vrtti nirodha.
Yoga is the intimacy that's left when there is no (mis)-identification with the elaborations of the mind.[1]

But the elaborations of the mind don't stop forever; thinking never comes to an end. What happens is that when we see our mental elaboration and stories as just conceptions, we no longer identify with them. When we practice this kind of watching and feeling all day long on retreat, it's much easier to work with the mind states that naturally and relentlessly arise in daily life. There is no separation between formal practice and daily life. While you sit here now, this is daily life. And later this week, when you sort through your e-mails, this is also formal practice.

We can understand this nonseparation we call Yoga by studying the life of the almonds we've been eating at break. Almond trees are not self-pollinating; they require pollination through the activity of bees.

In California last year, I learned about the relationship between almonds and dairy. When the dairy cow population increased exponentially in the 1950s, so did the use of pesticides. The pesticides have been decimating the landscape ever since, and the primary casualty is the honeybee. And when the honeybee population declines, we see fewer and fewer almonds. It's an intimate relationship.

This practice of Yoga and Buddhism may reduce the ways we suffer individually and collectively, but it does not end desire. Desire is the creative heart of being alive. Sometimes we contract around what we desire and become attached to getting exactly what we imagine. Sometimes we *think* we need something that we later realize we don't. Certainly the way we meet desire determines whether we are going to suffer or not, but the desire to create, to change, to build, and to take apart is what keeps life meaningful. We are never beyond action.

There is no intimacy in maintaining a life that is always conceptual, always relating to things through our knowledge base. It is curiosity and desire that give rise to intimacy. So that's why we practice. Our motive may change, our circumstances may change, but at bottom, we all desire a certain kind of intimacy that is healing and energizing. This is why we practice. This is also why our practice is so important in times of economic and ecological imbalance.

In practice, as in much of the early Vedas, there is a constant tuning of attention to the natural world. The following lines describe the way attention (the spirit of energy, the energy of spirit) tends to become extroverted and lost to the inherent intimacy of reality. These words are like a prayer, or even a wake-up call in these troubled times. I like to imagine that the word *spirit* means our attention span.

> If your spirit has gone to the four corners of the world far
> away, we turn it back so that you can dwell here, now.
> If your spirit has gone to the billowy ocean far, far away, we
> turn it back so that you can dwell here, now.
> If your spirit has gone to the flowing streams of light far
> away, we bring it back so you can live here, now.
> If your spirit has gone to the waters, or to the plants, far
> away, bring it back so you can live here, now.
> If your spirit has gone to the sun, or to the dawns far away,
> we turn it back to you here to dwell and live.
> If your spirit has gone to the high mountains far away, bring
> it back so you can live here, now.
> If your spirit has gone to what has been and what is to be,
> far away, we turn it back to you to dwell and live.[2]

Flesherton, Ontario, September 2008

15

End of Retreat

Days and nights, in walking, standing still, sitting and
lying down, if you always contemplate in this way, you
will know that your own body is like the moon in water, the reflection in a mirror, the heat waves in a hot
day, the echo in the empty valley. You cannot say it is
a being because even if you try to catch it you cannot
see its substance. You cannot say it is non-being either
because it is clearly in front of your eyes.
—DOSHIN, *Ryoga-sijiki*

L AST NIGHT AFTER our final meditation session, as I walked
out of the hall, I looked back at the cushions lined up in rows
and felt all the hard work and also the quietness of the day. My
breathing was easy. When I walked outside I felt a longing to turn
around and sit back down for the rest of the night. As we end retreat,
notice where the energy wants to move for you—forward into the
world or hanging on to the peaceful silence of retreat—and see if
you can continually attend to each arising moment and shift over
and over again into each new situation.

I am interested in supporting a Yoga practice that is concerned
with the day-to-day life of people who are not going to spend their

years in monasteries or wandering through forests and river deltas. Although I recommend monastic practice and forest dwelling wherever appropriate, monks are not the population I work with primarily. I want the practices we explore to be on a par with what is possible in our everyday lives. This doesn't mean that we can just adopt practice that "fits in" to our lifestyles. If the practices are to be vibrant and challenging, they must also interrupt the habits of everyday domestic life. The Buddha is said to have once remarked that "a house gathers dust."

Practice can't be divorced from the social world. *Samādhi* is a meditative awareness that is brought on through wholehearted practice of *dhāraṇā* (concentration on an object of meditation) and *dhyāna* (absorption and stillness). I interpret *samādhi* as the realization of the inherent intimacy of all things. It is the *teleos* of formal meditation practice. *Samādhi* does not just occur in one instant. It actually provides an ongoing and unshakable way of looking at the world. Also, the feeling of oneness that characterizes deep meditative absorption is impermanent. The experience is transitory. The wisdom may be unshakable, but the actual stillness that occurs in *samādhi* is not eternal—it does not continue indefinitely. We have to get up, pee, and make lunch. We have to take action. Stillness without action is only *samādhi* in drag.

There are no hermetically sealed practices or cultures. Now that cultures are flowing into and out of one another at a dramatic pace, there is nothing more radical than being silent. Stay at home for a while. Sit under trees. Serve. Study. The whole idea of what it means to be a person is so radically challenged by these practices. Through meditation practice we cultivate a specific quality of awareness—it is nonjudgmental, and it has a quieting effect on the inner body. I continue to cultivate this quality of mind (knowing that is always behind the fluctuations of thought anyway) so that I can be in life with more vividness and stability, and less distractedness and expectation.

Note the following passage from the *Tao Te Ching:*

The sage dwells in affairs of nonaction [*wu wei*]. . . . He acts but does not presume; he completes his work but does not dwell on it.[1]

Likewise in the Bhagavad-Gītā:

For there is no person on earth who can fully renounce living work, but one who renounces the reward of work is in truth a person of renunciation.

When work is done for a reward, the work brings pleasure or pain or both, in its time, but when a person does work for work's sake, the work is simply his or her reward.[2]

There is always work to be done, to be sure, but action without clinging is the heart of karma Yoga. When making music, writing, or even making love, nondoing means letting go of our *mental preoccupation* with a goal. In this way, our activity does not have a dramatic bearing on our self-image or self-esteem.

The value of an action lies completely with itself even though its effects ripple everywhere. In other words, action in the karma Yoga perspective can be clear and purposeful, but we cannot control the outcome. Every action is a moment of practice, an expression of intimacy, an expression of one's self. Dogen wrote, "When one [who is enlightened] has seen an exhausted turtle or an ailing sparrow, one doesn't want their thanks—one is simply moved to helpful action."[3]

The practice of meditation not only helps the clarity of our perception but can also build our moral character. Meditation cannot guarantee some kind of virtuous life, but it can certainly prepare the ground for ethical wisdom. In the simplicity of silence, most people can feel their delusions and obsessions softening.

Of course we must also remember that yogic *samādhi* is nothing special. All kinds of people enter into *samādhi* all the time without knowing anything about it. We just happen to be doing this practice of body and mind. But some gardeners, for instance, are just in it, just doing their work; maybe they don't think about it all that much!

Even though history is infinite, we can only know history in the present. And we shape our dispositions by the way we meet them. In everything we do, we are choreographing our electric brains and the cultural-biological grooves we leave behind. Our actions matter. The way we perceive each moment matters, because how we perceive something determines the way it's conditioned.

Practice starts where you are and ends where you are. You can't practice ahead of or behind yourself. Your "self" is the manifestation of the natural world right here and right now. How can you know where it begins and ends? Patañjali describes change in this way: "Being delivered into a new form comes about when natural forces overflow."[4]

Picture a river rushing up against a fallen log: a new form comes about when the natural world pushes a form forward. This is happening over and over again in each consecutive moment. The exhale completes itself at *mūla bandha,* and then there is a natural pause where the toning of the pelvic floor receives the exhaling patterns and then springs up in its center with an inhale. The inhale is born in the pause that completes the exhale. Likewise when you die—this happens on an exhale—the body begins deteriorating and returning to the earth. Whether it is burned or buried or left to the birds, the elements that make up this body continue into new form. What happens to the "I-maker" is unknown from our standpoint. But we know that the material body shifts into new form.

Our personal life might come to a blurred close with our final exhalation, but the great breath keeps moving. The *spanda* (vibration) keeps pulsating: the toe is eaten by a worm that is eaten by a bird that is eaten by a larger bird that flies over the same valley in which we are sitting. Look up at the birds circling the hills today—they are made of the very stuff we are. We could never draw an accurate map of this process. We can never really see the underground rivulets that bring water to the well. But we can feel the process of change in everything we do. The underground rivers thundering beneath our feet, the ongoing movements of inhaling and exhaling, the changing expression or complexion of your face as you listen to these words—this is the ground of reality, this is the ground of Yoga.

The *Heart Sūtra* says, "Form is emptiness, emptiness is form."[5] You can't tell one from the other. You can't separate them and say, "This is my self, and this is the breath." The breath is the self; the self is the vast sky and river and mind. The breath can't leave the sky, the *spanda* is not separate from the mind or the tree or language. Again, the basis for our discontent and distortion lies not in a world "out there" but in our skewed perceptions. "To authentically solve the problem," Stephen Batchelor teaches, "it is necessary to turn our attention away from the task of struggling with a stubborn and intractable world and to turn it instead to dispelling the ignorance that mistakenly causes such a world to appear."[6] We don't have to strain in our effort to right the world—we just have to clarify our ways of seeing.

When you practice the Yoga postures, you don't need much theory: just step into them. The energy of the body and the vast array of sensations change, and as they change we move right into them, become them. We move through the posture into the posture, so to speak. We move beyond the form of the posture with the mind so that our ideas about the pose drop away. If you push away certain feelings, you get attached to them. There is no final end point for the Yoga posture. It's never complete. It's more like a little path that over distance dwindles into nothing in the forest. The path becomes the forest. The posture techniques become something much larger than a Yoga pose. When you find some discomfort, just immediately open to it. So, instead of closing down, you just get bigger.

When I work with my body, I am working with that aspect of reality. When I watch my mind and its complications and speed, I am watching that aspect of reality. When I wash my body, I am washing the universe.

But if I am the same as the universe, you might wonder why you're all on that side of the room facing me, alone here in this part of the room. This seems to be the form we've set up. It's conducive to dialogue, but it supports a kind of duality as well. If we are getting bigger, which we could interpret as the awareness encompassing everything, then why not adjust the rituals here and the layout of the room so that its more conducive to a nonhierarchical approach?

Maybe we could parallel the open source model: everything is flat, available, open for interpretation. We can lay these practices out for all to learn and then talk together about what works and what doesn't. Community awakening rather than personal awakening. Even when we study a river, we come to find that it flows both ways.

Sherwood Park, Alberta, 2010

16

The Nonduality of Inner and Outer Practice

Intimacy is not identifying with the elaborations of the mind.
—Patañjali, *Yoga-Sūtra 1.2*

THERE ARE EIGHT limbs of Yoga that constitute Patañjali's Raja Yoga.[1]

1. *Yama* (external restraint): the clarification of one's relationship to the human and nonhuman world.

2. *Niyama* (internal restraint): personal principles governing the cultivation of insight, including *śauca,* purification; *santoṣha,* contentment; *tapas,* discipline, patience; *svādhyāya,* self-study, contemplation; and *īśvara-praṇidhāna,* devotion, aspiration, and dedication to the ideal of pure awareness.

3. *Āsana* (posture): cultivation of profound physical and psychological steadiness and ease in mind, breath, and body. Practice of Yoga postures.

4. *Prāṇāyāma* (breath and energetic regulation): sustained observation and relaxation of all aspects of breathing, bringing

about a natural refinement of the mind-body process through the stilling of the respiratory process.

5. *Pratyāhāra* (withdrawing of the senses): a naturally occurring uncoupling of sense organs from sense objects as awareness interiorizes.

6. *Dhāraṇā* (concentration meditation): locking awareness on a single object (e.g., sound, breath, sensations in the body) until the field of awareness becomes singular and focused.

7. *Dhyāna* (absorption): concentration deepens to the point where subject and object dissolve and the sense of "me" is temporarily absent.

8. *Samādhi* (integration): the sustained experience of concentration where there is a complete integration of subject and object, revealing pure awareness and interconnectedness.

When I begin working with students who want to establish a well-rounded practice, we always begin with the first limb of practice, the *yamas,* as a means of setting a foundation for what spiritual practice means and how it ripens in contemporary life. This approach helps dismantle our lofty associations to the term *spiritual* so that practice begins grounded in the material. When we begin with the five *yamas,* our Yoga practice grows roots in the intricate and infinite web of living relationships and thus presses the Yoga practitioner not to turn away from the world but to tune in to and be tuned by the life of relational existence. How we relate to ourselves, other humans, plants, animals, architecture, city planning, the growing of food, and the daily tasks in the household are all part and parcel of the path of Yoga practice. Sometimes people are not sure how to begin a practice or even how to mature a practice once they've begun. This list is not just sequential—it gives us an overview of the varied elements that constitute a path. Although we use these lists as suggestions, how they manifest in a unique life looks very different for each individual and community.

The formal personal practice of *āsana, prāṇāyāma,* ethics, and *samādhi* is fundamental to the Yoga path, and a practice engaged with everyday life rests upon the insight that we must begin to change ourselves before we can help to change the world. Out of such an approach, some conclude that it is enough to foster change on an individual level. Society is an aggregate of individuals, and if enough individuals change, then so will society as a whole. You are a corner of culture. Society, however, is more than an aggregate composition of individuals. People create society, but social structures also create (socialize) people. It is a kind of feedback loop without beginning or end. What is radical about this practice is that we can work on the personal and institutional simultaneously.

When I see that the habitual drives of attachment and aversion or the mental states of greed, envy, competitiveness, anger, and confusion are potentials within my mind-body, I recognize that karma works through me in every moment. In each moment, my perception and action may be informed by the momentum of these negative energies. When I look into my family or community or political culture, I see so much intolerance and inflexibility. Inward and outward, I can easily see the vivid manifestation and acting out of these energies.

Karma reminds us that our actions have an effect, but it also reminds us that our intentions are informed by our belief systems. A Yoga practice is always engaged with the world. It cannot be any other way, because my actions always have an effect.

When I work with my capacity for anger and intolerance, I am working on the mind, body, and society because I'm not planting seeds of aggression or indifference. Not acting out anger in harmful ways to myself or others takes care of my anger so that it isn't flowing through the culture. In this way my "inner" work is also "outer" work because I'm a corner of culture. When the mind is less pulled by these deep patterns of clinging, I can also see how the patterns operate in others, operate in institutions, and then how those aspects of culture influence my own mind stream.

Action is the key to Yoga because it recognizes the deep interrelatedness of all things. This is the relationship between karma and *samādhi*. Causality demonstrates intimacy. The background of anything is everything.

Wisdom (*prajñā*) is the maturation of insight. When we gain insight into the workings of our own minds, we can begin to take action from a clearer perspective. The real purpose of practice is to discover the wisdom that springs up in each and every moment. Discovering yourself is to discover wisdom; without discovering yourself you can never communicate with anybody or see anything clearly. Saying someone made you angry is not intimacy: it's blame, it's projection. We can be intimate with anger. We can be intimate with sadness. We can be intimate with hurt and even rage. Intimacy means opening to what is without necessarily acting it out or turning it in. When we sigh and allow the attention and breath to soften into a relaxed pattern, it feels as if some rusty old hasp gets unlocked, and we slowly open past the limits of fear and habit. To simply open to what is coming alive in each and every moment is intimacy. Practice gives us practical skills so we can move out of our unconscious identification with the content of awareness. Acting out anger is actually a way of making the ego more comfortable. Pushing away anger is a form of denial. So the skill and wisdom of practice is to pursue the middle path, settling into our own nature. This includes the whole parade of emotions and thoughts that moves through us, yet without identification, blame, or acting out. A feeling is something in your body. So how can you separate your stories from what your feelings are? The stories are just our way of rationalizing and justifying what we're feeling. We also use our stories to avoid feeling what we're feeling, seeing what we're seeing. Allen Ginsberg couldn't have said it better:

> Talk when you talk
> Cry when you cry
> Lie down when you lie down
> Die when you die[2]

Seeing clearly is called *vidyā,* from the root *vid,* or *video:* to see. It's not that we gain special powers or completely objective visions but that we can begin to see the way things happen, the way things come to be. This is nonduality, this is affinity. So when we say that the original nature of mind is nondual, what are we actually talking about? As soon as you think you've accomplished nonduality, you have to let go of *that* because that can become a fixed position, and that's not intimacy. When the heart is open, there is really nothing left to say!

Copenhagen, Denmark, 2006

17

Money and the
Turnings of Mind

It is quite obvious that without material progress we
will lack many material comforts. In the meantime,
without inner peace material things alone are not sufficient. There are many signs which indicate that material progress alone is not sufficient. There is something
lacking. Therefore, the only way is to combine the
two.
—THE FOURTEENTH DALAI LAMA, UNIVERSAL
RESPONSIBILITY AND THE GOOD HEART

NOBODY TALKS about money as a spiritual practice. We
barely talk about money in our everyday lives. I want to talk
about money.

Human beings need the freedom to work at meaningful jobs.
Part of the teachings on "right livelihood" mean endeavoring to
take up work that does not exploit or kill. We work as a form of
service. When I first studied Zen Buddhism, I was handed a sheet of
paper at the temple with the instruction for carrying out practice in
my workplace. I still have the page. It reads:

Right Livelihood deals with the five kinds of trades that should be avoided by a lay disciple. They are:

trade in deadly weapons
trade in animals for slaughter
trade in slavery
trade in intoxicants
trade in poisons[1]

Right Livelihood means earning one's living in a way that is not harmful to others.

Reflecting on these principles now, they seem to capture what it means to have a livelihood integrated into one's practice. This is appropriate livelihood. Yoga and Buddhist teachings are not serving us well—and neither are any spiritual "schools"—if they do not tie together our contemporary forms of work and consumerism with deep values like community, generosity, and friendship. The great religious traditions need to remind us that external forms of wealth simply don't ground us in the way we think they will. If we use savings accounts and retirement plans as the solution to our unhappiness, this will only lead to greater degrees of dissatisfaction and craving. Traditional societies even in the recent past made fewer distinctions between the economic, social, and religious spheres. Modern interconnectedness is going to bring this to the surface again. We can no longer act in ways that try to safeguard our individual security (or greed) at the expense of others and the natural world. Greed is simply part of a defective value system. This is based on an erroneous belief that the self is a separate entity. I try to recognize my own complicity in this system, not only through what I consume, but also through the effects that the funds in my bank account have upon the workings of the market.

In the way I live my life I strive to uproot the momentum that greed has on me personally. I struggle with my desires every day. I do my best to live simply.

Our secular cravings have created a system that can never satisfy itself. It is symptomatic of a spiritual need that cannot be met through the market. Maybe the solution to these enormous ecological and economic imbalances is simply to recognize that they are a mirror of what is going on in all of us, and until those repressed needs for connection and simplicity are met, we will continue acting in harmful ways. Yet what we know about repression is that eventually that which is repressed will find a way forward. For the time being, however, that means fighting against a system that is, at bottom, a false religion.

The market system allows humans to realize their innate capacity for creative expression, but it also serves those whose entrepreneurial skills can easily get mixed up with self-interest. I am not an economist, but I'd like to begin a conversation about money and the markets so that we can include all aspects of our lives—even economic—in our practice and community dialogue.

No matter how advanced and interesting our urban lives, we never live too far from those who grow our food, tend the land, and protect biodiversity. It is only in knowing deeply the links in the ecological chains of interbeing that we can live a life of felt connection to the earth, ourselves, and each other. Patañjali's iron age was very different from the world in which we find ourselves today. Westerners who approach Yoga live in a very different culture, an intensely individualistic culture with a social milieu utterly different from that in which the teachings originated.

While Patañjali deals with the aspects of our minds that are universal, such universality is always in action in a cultural milieu. We cannot focus on the universal principles of our human beingness without taking into account the context of that human's life. This presents us with the challenge of engaging in our practice with great commitment while also exploring teachings with critical engagement. Putting theory and practice together and applying both in daily life makes Yoga alive.

In 1486, in his *Oration on the Dignity of Man,* Italian Renaissance philosopher Pico della Mirandolla proclaimed the arrival of the free, self-defining individual, starting the trend to individual rather than collective sensibility.[2] Three hundred years later the Rights of Man were proclaimed, bringing the end of an ancient culture of communally rooted responsibilities. The collective virtues of acceptance, humility, and restraint rapidly disappeared. We think of the human perspective as dominant.

In the widening split between private and public, state and church, individual and collective, mind and body, nature and culture, the self began to emerge as the central player in the greater web of social and economic life. In the present era, the overvaluation of individualism is associated with personal alienation. This has increasingly and exponentially characterized the past one hundred years of Western culture. In the search for ever-greater individual freedom, we have dissolved all those personal, social, and ecological restraints, reciprocities, and responsibilities that were the sources of collective support and security. Eco-social crisis and the widespread crisis of personal identity and meaninglessness are ultimately one and the same. Alienated individuals seek an intensely individualistic spirituality with a functional sensibility, a spirituality that delivers on "fast food" expectations, and an obsession with material rewards or reifications that signify the achievement of enlightenment. This stubborn and rootless individualism makes community—even spiritual community—difficult for many of us. Unrestrained desire cancels, even annihilates community and relationship.

When attention to this moment is reduced to attention to "me" and "mine," we ruin the relations out of which we are born. Looking, listening, touching, and hearing the other is a radical path of intimacy. Radical love. The tender gesture of opening to the other is actually opening to ourselves, to this body, to this breath. We forget about ourselves, about hierarchical relations, and open a space between persons. In space new creative relationships can be built.

We may easily create distinctions between private and public, you and I, inside or outside, but at root, the mystery of life itself always fractures our categories. Such a mystery levels all categories and reminds us that dividing up life is a very human condition that ensnares even our best intentions. The more we perceive our personal lives to be separate from our work, our habits separate from our ecology, and our bodies separate from the very earth itself, the more we reify such separation.

We are suffering from a profound lack of imagination. If the mind can fall into habits of fragmentation so deeply ingrained and so unnatural to reality, surely our imagination can expand to include a much more realistic mode of living in which we conceive of ourselves as part of a fluctuating web, even if our insights are not fully matured.

If your wealth is made of gardens and relationships, then you can eat and live off your wealth. If your wealth is made of representational symbols, like money, its very hard to stay connected to the earth, to one another, to the value of your hands and feet and breath. The vulnerability of our economy right now has everything to with debt and the way we worship the god of money. We've imbued money with a representational value that has been so exaggerated that the system we've created no longer creates balance or community wealth.

There is also a tension in life between time and money. You can have a lot of money and no time. Without time there is little room for generosity and friendship. It's easier to create relational bonds in the sphere of time than in the sphere of money. I encourage practitioners who study with me and in our wider community to really meditate on voluntary simplicity so we have more time to focus on relationships, friendships, life. My friend David Loy said, "Money is something we have, but time is what we are."[3]

Money is a medium of exchange, but more subtly, it's a storehouse of intense value and fantasy. It's a collective agreement in which we all place our most intense fears. The fear of impermanence is hidden within our retirement accounts and the language we use around savings. This is not a fear of not being able to eat but a deeper fear about how unreal we are. I think that feeling part of a community helps tether our greed and self-centeredness. So does the kind of practice that keeps us in touch with the body and the earth. I teach Yoga as an ethical mind-body-community practice that returns us to relational life, so we do not fall into the vortex of the egoic power that comes from the me-dominated view. When our attitude toward money is overloaded with greed, it's injected with self-centeredness. Community practice helps undo this.

So often we think that spirituality and money do not belong together. If religion is a realm devoted to the beyond, it may not have much to say about money. When we turn our spiritual practice toward this world at this time, then money can be included in our practice. Spiritual teachings and teachers—communities on the whole—should not be silent on the matters of profit, loss, and economic distribution. If we are not supposed to lie and cheat, shouldn't we also have an ethics about money? We are spiritual, corporeal, and also economic creatures. How can these be divorced?

Markets are not "good" or "bad." They are both good *and* bad. Markets can benefit and enrich the lives of the poor and generate new jobs and support talent. They can also displace huge sectors of society and disempower those who don't have mainstream skills. The role of Yoga philosophy and practice here is not antimarket or promarket. It aims at the underlying psychology of greed and delusion. If a market network is always made of individuals, and we must remember that if a market is a true democratic realm, then its focus is on relationships. So the key question is not are we for or against the capitalist marketplace, but rather do we understand what the limits are to free markets as the organizing structures of our lives? We must balance our self-interest and individualistic motivations with a loyalty to community. We need to look deeply at personal and institutionalized forms of greed.

It is hoped that this dialogue about "right livelihood" can merge with the work of those in the nonspiritual sector who aim to think about community interests as well as individual interests. As yogis we need to look outside our field to converse with those who understand the economy very well. The answer is not going to come from one side. We must learn how to redistribute resources for those who cannot achieve economic self-sufficiency in the market alone. We need a social and ecological vision of money so that we are not blind to effects of our actions in the marketplace. We need an economic vision that guarantees that the basic needs of every person are met and satisfied.

The power of the market model rests on the assumption that markets work best when left entirely on their own—this is how efficient competition is achieved. We buy goods at the lowest possible price to sell them at the highest. This achieves efficiency, incentives for productivity, and a level of activity that needs no central direction or organization. No one buyer and seller can have absolute market reign. Of course, this is a very simplistic description of our economic model. But the key point is that the market language is geared toward thinking that better or worse can be measured by more or less. More choice is better, more goods are better, and more capital is better. Yet Yoga reminds us, through *aparigraha* (nonacquisitiveness) and just about every other teaching, that we also need to be "other oriented." Other, in this case, also refers to city planning. It refers to fish, rivers, and the air. Self-interest is not an adequate faith. With such an attitude, more is not better. Spiritual life cannot be separated from economic transactions. In fact, *spiritual life* is a misnomer, a holdover term that does not adequately describe our commitment to the material. The yogi is a materialist in the best sense of the word—one who loves and cares for the material. My understanding of *spiritual* is to be deeply engaged in the material.

The Christian paradigm has always had a concern for the poor and a care for those who have greater needs. I have always read the Bible's key message as "God is with the poor in their struggle." The self-interest model of economic exchange must be balanced with some kind of "other-interest" practice in order to nurture the diversity of our social and economic webs.

The global reach of the market makes our neighbors quite close to us. The environmental cost of excessive growth is just too high. The personal costs of self-interest are also too high. Some of the worst cases of environmental degradation from industry happened in the Soviet Union under centrally regulated, nonmarket economic conditions. It's not correct to simply blame free markets: we need to look inward at our own ethical commitments, our sense of connectedness to a wider whole, and our sense of community as well.

Voluntary simplicity is one example of how we can change our economic conditions. Voluntary simplicity is also a great way to teach our children about what matters and what we most value. Simplicity carves time out of busy schedules so we can enjoy friendship and balanced health, providing a means to redistribute our own abundant resources with others who lack the chance. I am very skeptical of romantic notions of back to the land and subsistence farming. I have seen what it's like to live in poverty in rural areas that are not part of the wider economic trading system. It's not so romantic.

Like secular or creative ability, wealth itself is not bad. It can be used in many ways. But not all of the population has benefited equally from market and economic expansion, so we must look underneath wealth for the greed and fear that turns wealth into a powerful weapon. The role of the Yoga community, the *sangha,* is not to be for or against capitalism—it is life affirming. Valuing diversity, we must speak out against forces that oppress and exploit, and we must look inward at our own capacity to do the same. We need a framework or a language that allows members of the community and citizens at-large to grasp the values that the market ignores or sidelines.

Ethics can be a practice of creativity. What's interesting about the *yamas* (nonviolence, honesty, not stealing, wise use of energy, and nongreed) is that sometimes we really need rules and sometimes what's most important is the soul of those commitments. Rules can be guidelines for awakened action, where tenderness and community come before self-interest.

There are times when other-interest is more important than self-interest. A society needs to respond more effectively to the human pain caused solely by market outcomes. Our freedom to have choices at the supermarket or car dealership must give way to deeper values. Otherwise we miss out on the most nourishing aspects of our lives. We miss life. We become fragmented by greed, ill will, and the confusing messages of consumer culture. Living in a dazed state of greed is like confusing the moon for a porch light left on all night.

Crete, 2006

PART FOUR

Grounded in the World

18

Activism with Both
Feet on the Ground

We believe that all relationships . . . can be renewed by
restoring the pathways to connection.
—JEAN BAKER MILLER AND
IRENE PIERCE STIVER

WE HAVE DISCUSSED the importance of the *yamas* as an
ethical foundation for practice, and we've seen that the *yamas*
are an expression of interconnectedness and nonduality. Ongoing
practice is important as we open our eyes not only to our personal
forms of discontent but to the suffering of the world, moving syn-
chronistically along the parallel paths of inner and outer practice.
What we need to aim for is a creative activism grounded in wisdom
and morality, inclusiveness and community, and an integral practice
grounded in the recognition that there is no separation. On previous
retreats we've explored the *yamas* as detailed suggestions that together act as stages on the path of awakening. This is a helpful way of
working with the *yamas* at certain phases of practice and for different kinds of people. But remember that the *yamas* are also natural
expressions of human action, and that no one single path guarantees

the truth. If we turn the term *Yoga* into too much of an idealistic state or utopian achievement, we will fail to see the intimacy of all things right here in our imperfect culture, aging bodies, distracted minds, and everyday challenges.

Sometimes activists are burned out. Sometimes we don't take care of ourselves. In any relationship or long-term service, care and inspiration are dependent on staying connected with one's life force. If we are not connected to what makes us feel alive, our work and relationships begin to suffer no matter how "good" they are. "Not self" or "emptiness" does not mean the self does not exist. It means nothing belongs to the self in the way we think it does. But to look at ourselves in this way, we need to be in a place that is grounded and balanced. To serve others in a way that recognizes interconnection, we need to take care of ourselves. When we realize interdependence, we take better care of our bodies. When we realize interdependence, we take better care of others. The same goes for the earth, our cities, and our lives.

In the political sphere, government and nongovernment agencies often get too caught up in policies to pay adequate attention to their initial service mission. Programs suffer from frequent leadership turnover. Corruption often seeps into large organizations. The job of the *sangha* is to add a much-needed balance to the larger community as a whole. Balance comes from putting our practice to work in our families and communities and at the same time engaging in dialogue with those at the forefront of public issues. Yoga philosophy alone cannot deal adequately with the complexity of contemporary problems. Yogis must work with those who have expertise to solve the imbalances in their communities. We live in a modern economy— some of the core values of our practice are at odds with economic forces and values. This "going against the stream" provides a real benefit to the momentum of our societal habits.

Rather than thinking of transcendence as vertical, in Yoga, transcendence is horizontal. There is not a me that goes up or away or beyond but a collapse of that notion of "me" that puts the practitioner square in a relational field. I don't leave the body, I move through it. I don't leave the world, I find reality within it.

Too much anguish makes practice and action impossible. When caught up in distress and anxiety, Patañjali suggests we find renewed vitality and balance by cultivating benevolence to others and ourselves or making contact with the breath. Returning to the breath and its patterns returns us to the ground of the body, encouraging the basic gentleness in all of us to come to the foreground. Listen to how kind and nonaggressive Patañjali's advice is for working with habits, energies, and obstacles:

> Sickness, apathy, doubt, carelessness, laziness, hedonism, delusion, lack of progress, and inconsistency are all distractions from intimacy that, by stirring up consciousness, act as barriers to stillness.
>
> When they do, one may experience distress, depression, or the inability to maintain steadiness of posture or breathing.
>
> One can subdue these distractions by working with any one of the following principles of practice:
>
> Consciousness settles as one radiates friendliness, compassion, delight, and equanimity toward all things, whether pleasant, or painful, good or bad.
>
> Or, by pausing after breath flows in or out.
>
> Or, by steadily observing as new sensations materialize.[1]

Return to the body, Patañjali advises, return to the gentle and simple movement of the breath. Or, return to the attitude of benevolence and goodwill. Return, he proposes, to a relational life that begins with acceptance and kindness. Meeting conflict becomes a practice of nonaggression. The important point is that having kindness toward turbulent feeling in our minds or uncomfortable sensations in our bodies does not depend on qualities or changes in the discomfort itself. It depends on our own mode of perception. Likewise, kindness toward our enemies does not depend on any qualities in them but on our own generosity, patience, and capacity for sustained attention.

Even the ground we are standing on is undergoing constant flux. Our bodies, minds, and the earth itself are presently and continually undergoing relentless and sophisticated change. "When we behold a wide turf covered expanse," writes Darwin on the life of worms,

> we should remember that its smoothness, on which so much of its beauty depends, is mainly due to the inequalities having been slowly leveled by worms. It is a marvelous reflection that the whole of the superficial mould over any such expanse has passed, and will again pass, every few years through the body of worms . . . The plough is one of the most ancient and valuable of man's inventions; but long before he existed the land was in fact regularly ploughed, and still continues to be thus ploughed by earthworms. It may be doubted whether there are any other animals which have played so important a part in the history of the world, as have these lovely organized creatures."[2]

Like mind, breath, and body, the earth maintains itself through an ongoing process of change. Nowhere in the earth can we find some kind of soil or particle that is separate from this grand and often unseen process of change and relationship. There is no earth without this relationship and no worm without earth. Yet with our minds, we can create the illusion of separateness just as easily as we can see a lawn without worms.

Darwin's insight is this: when we look beneath the surface of what at first appears substantial and permanent, we find nothing other than "organized" relationships on which "beauty depends."

When you have insights like this about the relationship between the worm and the earth, the breath and the mind, our moods and the body, there comes a trust in the complexity of life—a trust with ground more solid than faith in one's own ideas about self and reality. Spiritual awakening comes with trust in something greater than one's own perception. We are all looking for this authentic connection to something living and large.

Once we are grounded in nonaggression and working from a place of relationship and trust, we can begin to conceptualize our next steps. The Natural Step is a Swedish organization (Det Naturaliga Steget) founded by researcher Dr. Karl-Henrik Robèrt in 1989. Its purpose is to teach and support environmental-systems thinking in corporations, cities, government, unions, and academic institutions through an easily understood dialogue that is rooted in basic science.

The Natural Step teachings are a series of sequenced scientific principles that provide a remarkable and comprehensive basis for understanding the requisites for life on Earth. In particular, it shows how individuals, organizations, and companies can act so that those requisites are maintained and enhanced. The purpose is to create real understanding of ecological connections without reducing the whole to a collection of details, disagreements, and counterarguments.

There are four "system conditions" that underlie the Natural Step and support the premise that every unique person is a "genius" in his or her own particular field. If individuals are supported, they can do a far more efficient job promoting change and harmony than any one final ideology. The four system conditions are as follows:

1. Nature cannot withstand a systematic buildup of dispersed matter mined from the Earth's crust (e.g., minerals, oil, etc.).
2. Nature cannot withstand a systematic buildup of persistent compounds made by humans (e.g., PCBs).
3. Nature cannot take a systematic deterioration of its capacity for renewal (e.g., harvesting fish faster than they can replenish, converting fertile land to desert).
4. Therefore, if we want life to continue, we must (a) be efficient in our use of resources and (b) promote justice—because ignoring poverty will lead the poor, for short-term survival, to destroy resources that we all need for long-term survival (e.g., the rainforests).[3]

Because these steps are scientifically incontrovertible and consensually derived, they tend to be supported across many diverse communities. They have an empowering language rather than an overly dire one. The materialistic appetite of our egoic impulses forms the engine of our relational and environmental destructiveness. Why, when we have so much, are we still devouring the earth at alarming speed and competing with one another in our hunger for more?

The answer has two main dimensions. Part of the problem lies in the dynamic of our economic system; part lies in our psychological/ spiritual condition. Understanding both perspectives is necessary to illuminate the sources of our insatiability.

In *The Evolving Self,* Mihaly Csikszentmihalyi declares that the time of innocence is now past; it is no longer possible for mankind to blunder about self-indulgently. Our species has become too powerful to be led by instincts alone. Birds and lemmings cannot do much damage except to themselves, but we can destroy the entire matrix of life on the planet. The awesome powers we have stumbled into require a commensurate responsibility. As we become aware of the motives that shape our actions, as our place in the chain of evolution becomes clearer, we must find a meaningful and binding plan that will protect us and the rest of life from the consequences of what we have wrought.[4]

Since we are a planetary species, Csikszentmihalyi argues, such self-centeredness cannot continue. Until we move beyond personal identity as the sole motivation for action and begin to take in species identity or universal identity, ecological awareness will always be human centered. That is clearly not enough.

The only value that all human beings can readily share is the continuation of life on earth. In this one goal all individual self-interests are united. Unless such a species identity takes precedence over the more particular identities of faith, nation, family, or person, it will be difficult to agree on the course that must be taken to guarantee our future.[5]

Patañjali, from his post twenty-five hundred years ago, may help us articulate an empowering framework of values, virtues, and practices for individuals and communities. To bring Patañjali's teachings to life *now*, it's important to imagine him not as an all-seeing sage. He was a person (or even a group of people) responding to the psychological, existential, and social issues of the time. We can't divorce Buddha, Jesus, or any leading teacher from the condition of his or her time. How they responded to the imbalances of their particular society teaches us how we can respond to ours. This is the secular element of our practice.

It is precisely the actions we take as individuals that change the web of life for either better or worse. If the mind is like a vast field, the kind of seeds we plant in that field are up to us. If we plant seeds of harm and self-interest, greed and fear, those seeds will harvest in our communities, in our bodies, in our children, and in our landscape. If we plant seeds of compassion and equanimity, kindness and generosity, those energies will dominate in future harvests.

Such an attitude seeks partnership and solidarity and requires commitment on the part of practitioners to a life of nonharming and sensitivity. This calls for a rethinking of ethics within a vast framework of interconnectedness. We can then begin to feel awe as we embrace the 13.7 billion years of the unfolding universe through stars, galaxies, and even this very personal life-form. We are all made of stardust.

To treat others as we treat ourselves, a defining practice in most spiritual traditions, means that we are concerned for those on the other side of all of our transactions—even economic ones. We try our best to refrain from buying goods produced by workers who are impoverished or endangered by their work. We also try to choose livelihoods that value life. Over time I see that Yoga practices create a new sensibility in practitioners who undertake to make the dharma the core of their lives.

Although commercial Yoga studios have an important place in the modern marketplace, the traditions of Yoga long ago broke down institutional walls. Maybe today, Yoga will have to pierce through corporate walls. Even Krishnamacarya, a householder himself, valued the practice in terms of its contribution to the daily domestic life of both men and women. Though I am committed to practicing and sharing traditional teachings and forms, and though I continue to study with lineage holders in Buddhist traditions, I want to help free the teachings for their widest possible use throughout our society. Prisons, hospitals, and schools are *duḥkha* magnets. The dharma should be able to seep into every crack of our culture, supporting people who are suffering in body, heart, and mind.

I cannot find a hair's distance between issues of social justice, economic harmony, and the heart of the dharma: interdependence. To really embrace the heart of the world and stand up for it at the same time, the *sangha* we need most will be interfaith. There are so many Jewish and Catholic organizations doing great work around the earth. It's time for the yogis to organize in ways that cultivate a true yogic activism that embodies the great ideal of doing no harm and not living in ways that kill other life. A socially active and politically minded Yoga community can effect great social change if we partner with communities already doing important work.

As we build our Yoga communities to reach across ecumenical boundaries, we can begin offering established activist communities excellent tools for taking care of themselves and employing interdependent ethics within their organizations. The list of what the yogis can offer is endless and beyond the scope of this teaching, but these are simply words of encouragement so that we take this practice far afield and cultivate flourishing communities that begin with our own bodies and hearts.

Both Yoga and activism seem to flourish when they are practiced in a community. I always remind my students that we are not practicing to feel better or achieve something. We are practicing renunciation and devotion: renouncing our addictions and clinging and practicing devotion to a life of compassion and the welfare of all beings.

Training ourselves to stay focused and concentrated, especially on retreats and during longer periods of intense practice, helps create calmness and tranquillity in our everyday lives. Opening to the world, staying in tune with the breath, learning how to drop our viewpoint when necessary and express ourselves even when we feel terrified, are all factors that bridge the internal and external practices of Yoga. Tranquillity becomes the basic ground for taking action in a world that always requires our creative and grounded response.

In the *Vivekacūḍāmaṇi* of Śaṅkara, he says that the universe is "an unbroken series of perceptions,"[6] reminding us that from the perspective of Yoga it is only our minds that divide things up as "me" and "separate from me." That reality is composed of momentary events of sensation, feeling, thought, and perception is verifiable, and one does not need to accept this as an article of faith. Through practice and watching the movements of life within the field of awareness, we gain insight into impermanence and the truth that there is nothing that belongs to "me."

If there is nothing to hold on to, we begin to see that whatever is apprehended by the senses does not actually belong to them. With practice, the teachings of Yoga take on more and more significance because they can be tested out and verified. In our community, we always move back and forth between theory and practice so that our ideas remain rooted in personal experience rather than philosophical discourse.

We also encourage people to talk about their practice with each other so that they are honest about where they are. When you find something coming up in your practice, try to articulate it so that you can be sure to tend to it. You can begin allowing it into your own thought field, then maybe into a journal, then communicating with a friend. In this way community becomes a microculture where we are learning to support one another, which effectively makes Yoga a living tradition and not something of only exotic or antiquarian interest. While we are firm in our dedication to tradition through the preservation of practice and the study of our lineages, we are always experimenting and innovating.

We are so lucky that we can gather together as a community and practice in the tension of traditional teachings and contemporary

demands. Every form of Buddhism and Yoga is a hybrid of anteced-
ent practices within particular societies. Even the Buddha taught in
response to the political and social needs of his time. What is remarkable about the dharma is that it can emigrate from India and
China to Korea and Tibet and now the West and re-create itself in
response to the specific needs of those cultures. What we need is a
dharma that can respond to the militarism and consumerism that is
dominant in our world today and requires principles to live by (such
as equanimity and contentment) in order to supplant our addiction
to the three poisons: greed, hatred, and confusion. As globalization
intensifies worldwide social and environmental relations, there is no
way to avoid the karma of interconnectivity. Even my six-year-old
son wonders where the litter from his lunch will end up and why we
drive cars when we know we are running out of oil. Just today he
asked me if we can start biking to school all winter.

Our work in the dharma is taking the peace in our practice into
our communities and families and also our environment. This is
what I see as the heart of the dharma. People who truly practice any
spiritual tradition, regardless of geographical source, are also making
themselves into instruments of peace. At bottom, compassion is a
means of taking on the creative work of lessening suffering and turning the privilege of practice into a way of life that protects the rights
and lives of all beings.

What the Buddha taught as interdependence is exactly the same as
Patañjali's precept of not causing injury. What effects one molecule
of life effects all others indirectly. The *sangha* is not a community of
students revering a tradition or a teacher but a community that has
an allegiance to the welfare of all beings, rivers, winds, and arts. If
the dharma is not a challenge to militarism and consumerism, and if
it does not go deep into our own hearts to resolve the incessant hunger of desire, the dharma will just blend into pop values. But Yoga
and Buddhism are not products. They are not subservient to pop values and trends. This practice of working with our bodies and minds

can easily get neutralized in a culture that wants to turn everything into a product. But what is the function of a buddha?

Is a buddha one whose intention is to feel good? Or can the Buddha reorganize the internal and structural values of a society? From the other end of the spectrum, it is not enough to simply create social change; you have to wake yourself up in the process. *Duḥkha* is the inability to be creative and joyful. When we are stuck in our bodies and in our relationships, our society gets stuck. If we don't use the practices we learn, we just nourish this personal and social suffering. We have a great opportunity to foster an engaged, grassroots dharma that works both individually and culturally through which we can look at situations of suffering carefully, and for a long time, and then take loving action based on what we can see when we bring creative awareness to a situation.

This may sound like a simple recipe, but the work of opening to what's really going on inside and around us requires commitment and long-term practice. How can we live in a way where others are not being exploited at our expense? How can we build communities that can heal? How can we build a dharma that crosses ecumenical boundaries so that diverse groups can link up with each other?

At some level we all have resistance to practice. Some days I can't bear to walk through the gauzy snow in the dark morning light to go meet my *sangha*. But deep down, resistance to practice is resistance to change. A part of us does not want to let go. Over time, however, I have seen how this practice has helped me move through the world from a place of compassion rather than anger or apathy. What the dharma has to offer social activists and those in the medical and educational system is also a way to find meaning in our lives. Along with providing food, shelter, and security to marginalized people, we can also help them find meaning in their lives by connecting with others and learning about what nourishes them.

We are a collective experiment in awakening. In this way the guide for our actions is not based on whether something is pleasurable or self-satisfying but whether it is good for the whole and our place in it. Though this is not always easy, over time it is purifying. It also keeps the traditional teachings alive in contemporary culture and supports a Yoga practice engaged with this world, especially when we don't limit our definition of community to human beings alone.

Originally the word *secular* meant "at this time" or "of this age." It referred to the way a system comes alive in a particular context when it tunes in to the texture of its inimitable background. I suggest we aim for a secular Yoga that is alive and responsive to contemporary life, not an attempt at practicing exotic prayers and rituals that have no resonance or deep effect in our personal lives and commitments. We need a Yoga of *this* time.

Toronto, Ontario, 2007

19

The Lungs of the Earth

The *ṛṣis* and their culture were accompanied by farmers and their farms. Forest culture and farm culture. If you don't understand these two together, we are not going to get at the essence of Raja Yoga. When you turn to the aphorisms, the words will remain empty words.
—VIMALA THAKAR, *Hatha-Yoga*

CAN YOU HEAR the wind blowing through screens? That same wind is the breath in all of us. That same breath is in every bird and fish in this province and beyond. Today when we were digging out rocks from the garden, I wondered about the relationship between those worms in my fingers and the tiny imperceptible worms that live in the fauna of my intestines. How do worms breathe? Whenever the wind stopped this morning, I could hear all the leaves settle on the path. I imagined all the worms gathering small particles of soil into their ringed bodies and then burrowing down into their collapsing tunnels. Against the front window, I looked at the reflection of the garden, and all of us working in it, and I saw the breath being drawn into the nostrils of all of us and then trying to get out again. The wind doesn't really want to be inside us. It presses against the lung walls trying to escape again.

There were maggots in the compost. Or maybe they were some unrecognizable worm. When maggots crawl out of a decomposing corpse they die pretty soon. From the inside out, they break through the walls of the skin and die soon after. Maybe they can't live without a body to eat, without water, without blood? From time to time the wind stops right outside the window. Every time it does, I exhale. It's so quiet here. In the middle of a garden in the center of a city, it's quiet, and underground, it's so busy.

In the tales of the ascetics who set out on the path of awakening, the landscape, and the forests in particular, play a vital role in their practice. Turning away from the bustling towns and villages, the comfort of castles or of simple roofs, seekers moved into dense forests and wandered among the quiet trees and endless paths that meandered through uncharted landscapes. Gautama recalled his earliest childhood experience—playing in the shade under the canopy of a tree. The Buddha was later enlightened under a tree. He almost always offered his teachings under the shade of a tree, and he died under a wide canopy of leaves.[1] The medieval Yoga text *Yoga Vaśiṣṭha* describes the natural world with the precision of a poet, making it one of the central characters of its tales. The forest and the human body and imagination are seamless. Trees carry a serenity that is timeless. Trees protect the quiet and breathe along with us.

When you leave your favorite comforts and arrive on the first day of a workshop or retreat, you too are leaving the familiarity of what is known and continuing the ancient ritual of meaningful wandering. It's unfortunate that turning to the wild of the natural world is becoming more and more difficult. While the wild spaces of the human mind and body always remain, our forests are disappearing quickly. We need the forest canopies and the solid trunks of ancient trees in order to practice. This retreat is a treat for me because I'm not used to teaching students who are actively working with learning about and protecting the natural world. I will draw together the way these teachings and the research you're involved with dovetail.

The world is not made for us. I disagree with old translations of texts like *Yoga-Sūtra* and *Sāṃkhya Kārikā* that state that the world is only there for us to wake up. Who are we to say that the world was created for us, and when do the fish and grasses get a chance to state their claim?

The elements of earth, wind, air, and fire are integrated processes that make up the very fabric of our existence. They not only support our being alive, they truly make up the experience of life itself. Too often we think of ecological life as discrete organisms or bodies of water that somehow we need to return to in order to establish a more sustainable future. From a nondual perspective, it's not so much that we need to *return* to a relationship with the earth—we need to gain insight into the reality of *being* the earth in all of its manifestations. The earth is not mute. The earth is not a context or backdrop against which we live. Earth is synonymous with life. The earth and its organisms and minerals, winds and biodiversity, are resources that sustain and make up our very existence. Nonduality teaches us that Earth is not something that offers us resources and cargo, a passive "thing" that supports our activities. This mode of relating to the earth is not only dualistic but serves to turn resources into commodities.

I wish I could always feel how when I take a breath, every other creature is also taking a breath of the same air, even the trees. The incompressible breath, spreading through every forest and city in this very moment, connecting us all, unites us continually. Remembering the air in everything harmonizes any dissonance I'm feeling.

Rainforests cover 2% of the Earth's surface, or 1% of its landmass, yet they house over half the plant and animal species on Earth. They originally covered at least twice that area. Rainforests are being destroyed at a staggering rate. According to the National Academy of Science, at least 50 million acres a year are lost, an area the size of England, Wales and Scotland combined.

Despite the small land area they cover, rainforests are home to about half of the 5 to 10 million plant and animal species on the globe. Rainforests also support 90,000 of the 250,000 identified plant species.[2]

Think of the endless cycles of breath that move through our lungs, the constant regeneration of water and heat in our bodies, the return to the earth of everything we inhale and ingest. We are born of earth, sustained by earth, and return to earth even in each moment of experience. Yoga pushes our perceptual activities toward seeing and experiencing as a mode that is inverse to our habitual mode of separating causes and conditions. Humans are not above, superior to, or more important than Earth. In his essay "Endgame," Edward Hoagland writes:

> Blindly accelerating, we burn through entire galaxies of other life, unimaginably interlinked and unmapped—amputating ourselves from the rest of Creation, whether destroyed or still undestroyed. The risks are unfathomable. And if you don't find this tragic, open your heart.[3]

The restraints described as the first limb of Yoga practice continually turn us toward a more participatory and integrated experience of Earth and life. The *yamas* (ethics) are means of integrity that offer us a compelling mode of action that shifts our comprehension of nature from something centered around people to something that occurs with or without our human-centered perspective. The *yamas* are an essential step in protecting and perpetuating a nondual experience of nature. This redirects our actions by placing them in an ethical framework that begins from a place of nonseparation. Such an ethical framework places limits or restraints on our actions so that they are more fully integrated within the dynamics of how life functions in relationship rather than in isolation.

What is profound about the *yamas* in the context of ethical environmental responsibility is that they do not put human needs first. We see that there is no primary form of life that is more special than any other. Humans do not come before water any more than we can separate water from our bodies. If we continue to think of oceans as aquariums or the life of the earth as a terrarium, we will continually place the environment in the category of object that somehow supports or is at odds with our desires and needs as subjects. But whenever we create a separate thing, we find ourselves outside it. And a worldview whose axiom places humans at the center denies the very basis of human experience: nonduality.

Whenever we create *thingness,* whether personal, animal, system, or element, we turn what is a process into a conceptual category. This gives us the illusion that something can exist separate from the act of perception. *Life, ocean,* or *human* are linguistic categories that give us the feeling of separateness, because we confuse the category for the experience. When we name something, it begins to feel real. But Patañjali's teaching of *svarūpa śūnya* reminds us that at base there is no thing available in reality, rather there is simply the arising and passing away of experience.[4]

The yard outside my home is made of soil, water, air, worms, decomposing leaves, children's toys that are rusting beside a leaky garden hose, and bits of newspaper blown into a hole my son dug in the ground. The cycle of the yard and the growing and dying taking place cannot be boxed into units. It is a geosystem, a matrix, a continually occurring series of processes impossible to designate as this or that, impossible to separate into events or units. Organic and inorganic interact, creating an experience in the present moment of life unfolding.

This mode of seeing collapses the perceptual gap of a yard created by a "me" who enjoys the yard. The growth and death of the yard, like the cycles of inhaling or exhaling, is one of participation and change; all processes are living and dying and living again. My son's yellow Tonka tractor is rusting under the fence. The tractor has just as much dying in it as the leaves in the soil, and the new form the tractor is taking has just as much life in it as the garlic bulbs that are spreading their winter roots underground.

Experiencing these fundamental units, or what Patañjali calls the dharmas of experience,[5] means experiencing relationality. This means that we begin to experience life more clearly than language can. Each moment is called a *kṣaṇa*. We have this term in the Buddhadharma also. When the Buddha died, his teaching was codified into a philosophical framework called the Abidharma, in which most schools came to accept that time is made of moments (*kṣaṇavāda*). Although we can get carried away with trying to define and seize the infinitesimal, this view helped bring home the importance of seeing reality as a contingent and impermanent flow. Śaṇkarācārya actually challenged overreifying this theory of moments, because he said that if a moment is the smallest particle of time imaginable, how can the causal efficiency of that moment be made intelligible?[6] What he means is that although there is impermanence, we must not try to pin down what a moment actually is. Time is unable to be fixed and unable to die.

Buddhagosa's commentary on the Buddha's teaching attempts to capture impermanence clearly: "Just as the flame of a burning lamp, without leaving the area of the wick, breaks up then and there and when it burns or flickers in succession throughout the night it is called a lamp, even so, taking the succession [of states] this body is presented as enduring for a long time."[7] The seemingly established fact of a flame is nothing other than a moment-to-moment successive flow of contingent conditions. In the prereflective state of mind before ideas appear, we are one with time. When we see colors and shapes and feel tactile sensations, there is a flow with time in which we are not separating things out into this and that. Lived experience is an interwoven flow. Our practice aims to return us, over and again, to this very flow.

When we experience life in the context of life—as process rather than structure—what it means to be human becomes much wider and more global than our dualistic modes of perception allow. No matter where we look—the surface of the ocean, the earth's crust, the meeting of two human hands, or even two pairs of eyes—we find the interface of processes and the impermanent flux of earth, air, water, and life's ongoing diversity. If the organic and inorganic cannot be separated, if fish cannot live outside water, if human identity is made of relational existence, then thinking about *anything* means exploring life relationally. Humans not only exist in dependence on this earth but also have no hierarchical prominence in the scheme of life.

Ingrained cultural attitudes—the *saṁskāras* of the culture—have strong momentum. The closest we've come to dealing with the spiritual and psychological dimensions of collapsing ecological diversity is the deep ecology movement founded by Arne Naess. This deep, long-range ecology movement is based on a feeling for nature that sees the environmental crisis as a symptom of a psychological or spiritual ailment that afflicts modern humanity in technological societies.

We are enveloped by an illusion of separation from nature, made more extreme by human-first centeredness. Where Yoga and the deep ecology movement come together is not in terms of environmental action—that was unknown in Patañjali's day—but in the critique of the idea that we are the crown of creation and the measure of all beings. We tend to think that the world is a pyramid, with humanity rightly on top, and that nature is merely a resource. To maintain such a position, we have to cling to separation, security, and a fortified sense of self, all of which, according to the basic axioms of Yoga, create *duḥkha.*

What we cling to most, Patañjali cautions in the second chapter of the *Yoga-Sūtra,* is the attachment to a story of self.[8] This fundamental misperception is far more dangerous than biological warfare, sound pollution, contaminated water, or any chemical spills. What is most dangerous is that human beings think they belong to an order of being that can exist and should exist as separate from the living environment. Thinking that we exist as separate from each other is a case of mistaken identity. Deep ecologist Arne Naess writes:

"I am protecting the rainforest" develops into "I am part of the rainforest protecting myself. I am that part of the rainforest recently emerged into thinking." What a relief then! The thousands of years of imagined separation are over and we begin to recall our true nature.[9]

Naess's popular sense of deep ecology—what most people understand by this term—refers to the general idea of a nonanthropocentric or, more positively, an ecocentric approach to ecology/living-in-the-world. Whereas an anthropocentric orientation considers the nonhuman world as so many "resources" to be used as humans see fit, an ecocentric orientation attempts, within obvious kinds of practical limits, to allow all entities (including humans) the freedom to unfold in their own ways unhindered by the various forms of human domination.

Suppose that, to speak for the pine forests, we actually allowed ourselves to reexperience, to reapproach, the trees themselves. Then, after perhaps lifetimes of intimacy, we might be entitled to say something about what kind of relationship is possible and what ethical connection might or might not be demanded. Right now we are hardly able to begin to say.[10]

Ethics inspired not by law but by intimacy becomes a morality based on love. If I love the forests, I have a heightened sense of responsiveness and responsibility—not necessarily an ethic based on individual rights. Once again, we see that the *yamas,* from the perspective of *samādhi* (intimacy, integration, love) are not a matter of following rules or principles. It is action based on duty, commitment, and integration. Moral agency is a matter of deep insight, true self-being, genuine *samādhi.* Although morality is an innate human characteristic, ethics must be cultivated to bring such innateness to fruition. If the mind is always distracted and unable to settle in one place, it's impossible to have direct connection with what needs our attention. At this moment many of us would do well to still our mind by walking for few days in a dense forest. We need genuine contact with the natural world to *be* our natural world.

I have always been uncomfortable with the way that Yoga has been redefined in contemporary culture as not only a physical health regime but also a mainstream form of physical materialism. There is no doubt that Yoga postures and breathing practice are therapeutic. But cultivating a healthy body has become an obsession with youthful self-image and physical perfection. Look at the ways our culture has superimposed its values on Yoga practice. The commercial operation—and often the large profits that Yoga studios make—seems at odds with some of the basic values of Yoga: nonstealing, nonaccumulation, and the wise use of energy.

But beyond that there is a deeper issue, which is that Yoga has traditionally been *subcultural*. Yoga has always been a practice at the outskirts of culture because its practices had more to do with undoing habitual patterns than reinforcing the dominant grooves of the culture. As Yoga comes to the West, we need to look beyond the surface and investigate some of the basic axioms of practice not because there is anything wrong with a healthy body or a calm mind but because spiritual practice is always a practice of letting go rather than accumulation.

The academic needs to step out the door and have real time experience with what she studies. A father comes home from work and needs to connect with his child at play in a very different world than that of the office. We need to be present with each other and cultivate a mode of being that is living, wild, and direct. And unknowable, until it occurs.

Here is where many environmental and social theories fail: no matter how many new theoretical approaches we design to help us connect with the present moment, our momentum of habit, especially our habits of perception, interrupt our best intentions. This is where the path of Yoga is so important. Patañjali is not suggesting we take up ethics for ethics' sake, nor is he suggesting that only practicing restraints will bring satisfaction. Patañjali is more of a realist than an idealist—in his eight-limbed path he spends at least four limbs exploring meditation.

Without learning how to work with one's mind, there is no way to have direct unmediated, unfiltered experience. While going out into nature, hiking, making love, having intimate conversations, and having quiet time all offer forms of meditative experience, it is important to learn the skills necessary to interrupt the mind's continual patterns of dualistic perception. This begins in the body. The body is the best place to begin to reconnect with reality, because it is right here all the time. We need not make a pilgrimage any further than the felt body at this moment.

This is the magic of Yoga. One needs no props other than faith enough in the process each step of the way. This faith occurs just by going outside and sitting by trees, meeting others face-to-face, listening in conversation, and being present with whatever we are engaged in at that moment. This is not a nostalgic return to landscapes with trees and fields (although that is one part) but returning to our *true nature,* which is nothing other than what is occurring right now.

Nature is not external to us. Nature is not a product of natural sciences or an objective of organisms and organized systems but rather this very bodily existence. Death sets up our greatest ethical challenges because it moves us to see life structured by impermanence and interconnectedness. The human situation is that of birth and death and therefore we could say we are always being nature, nature unfolding. The unfolding task or journey of humanity or being human cannot be accomplished in isolation. In the essay "The Empirical Self," William James writes:

> The empirical self is all that he is tempted to call the name of "me." But it is clear that between what a man calls me and what he simply calls mine the line is difficult to draw. We feel and act about certain things that are ours very much as we feel and act about ourselves. Our fame, our children, the work of our hands, may be as dear to us as our bodies are, and arouse the same feelings and the same acts of reprisal if attacked. And our bodies, themselves, are they simply ours, or are they us?[11]

The point of ethical practice is that we are reaching out to listen rather than speak, to be touched rather than to touch, to be affected rather than to manipulate.

What is the logic of our destiny? We can't simply smile, return to our meditation cushions, and shut the door. This is an urgent call to practice!

Toronto, Ontario, 2009

PART FIVE

Encouragement and Conclusions

20

Suicide

No one ever lacks a good reason for suicide.
—Cesare Pavese

Most people come to contemplative practice because they've been hurt in some way. Many of us who have suffered trauma, pain, or existential loneliness have struggled to find stories to make sense of our lives. One of the challenges of cross cultural study—for example the interaction of Yoga, Buddhism, and Western psychological paradigms—is that it points out the shadows of the system to which we belong.

After many years of Yoga study, practice, and teaching, many of the assumptions I've held in my work as a psychotherapist have been brought to the surface—often in unsettling ways—through my struggle to integrate Yoga and Western psychology. While Yoga philosophy and Western psychology have much to learn from each other, what interests me is where they don't quite fit together smoothly. It's in these gaps between systems that we find fertile ground for exploration.

Yogic teachings on the fear of death (*abiniveśa*) have been very instructive in understanding the way we hold on to narratives about ourselves that reinforce and entrench feelings of alienation and suffering. While this is often readily apparent in others, it is also apparent in *my view* of others. Psychological diagnoses and pathology, while serving to help me recognize who and what I am working with, also serve to create separation in a space where intimacy is of paramount importance. Trying to be a good therapist or a helpful teacher can actually get in the way of healing.

One of my first psychotherapy patients was referred by a friend. He was a young man who was suffering from tremendous physical pain when symptoms from an old car accident reappeared after many years. Around the same time, one of his former boyfriends took his own life. "The two of these situations together," my colleague wrote to me, "have completely overwhelmed him. He wants to die."

My colleague made an appointment for him to see me because her own psychotherapy practice was full. "I'm not sure exactly what he needs," my friend told me. "Maybe a combination of listening and some practical tools like meditation so he can learn to accept what he is going through. Or maybe some medication or hospitalization."

The following Monday, at the time of our scheduled appointment, I waited for him and he never showed up. I left him a message and did not hear back.

One month later, I received a call from my friend who had referred him. She told me the man had taken his life. When I got the call I was stunned. I was in my first year of practice, and though I had never met this young man, I had imagined his walk, his face, his hair, his life. A feeling of relief came over me. I tried to distract myself from this strange response, but it surprised me. In the midst of this news, I was imagining that this man had found some relief.

When I was ten years old, our neighbor took her life. All I could do in response to her suicide was to visit "her" bridge every day for a year. After school, I'd ride my bicycle to where I imagined she had jumped, trying to envision what she thought about before she had leaped into the ravine below. I wondered if she noticed the bulrushes and the vast sky, the amazing view of the city or the beauty of the old trestle bridge.

When I was thirteen, I'd sit under the bridge for hours, smoking cigarettes, studying the deteriorating cement columns and rust leaking from the rebar through the cement railing. Three years after her death I continued visiting her last place on earth, her final view, her place of death. I couldn't let her go. It wasn't the loss of our distant friendship, my young crush on her, or my desire to see her pink bedroom again. I wanted to know what pushed her into such a singular view. How did she cross from an inner world of pain to the railing of the bridge? What in me held back that desire? What kept me from climbing that same railing?

The American photographer Diane Arbus ingested barbiturates and then cut her wrists with her razor; French painter Jeanne Hébuterne leaped from a third-story window two days after her partner, Modigliani, died of tuberculosis. She was pregnant with their second child. Mark Rothko took his life among his paintings; Spalding Gray, in the circling waters of the Hudson; John Berryman, jumping off a bridge in Minnesota; Anne Sexton, after visiting a hospital; and Virginia Woolf, weighing her pockets with stones and walking into the river near her home.

When preparing for this talk, I found this touching passage from Virginia Woolf in a letter to Leonard Woolf:

> I feel certain that I am going mad again. I feel we can't go through another of those terrible times. And I shan't recover this time. I begin to hear voices, and I can't concentrate. So I am doing what seems the best thing to do. You have given me the greatest possible happiness. You have been in every way all that anyone could be. I don't think two people could have been happier 'til this terrible disease came. I can't fight any longer. I know that I am spoiling your life, that without me you could work. And you will I know. You see I can't even write this properly. I can't read. What I want to say is I owe all the happiness of my life to you. You have been entirely patient with me and incredibly good. I want to say that—

everybody knows it. If anybody could have saved me it would have been you. Everything has gone from me but the certainty of your goodness. I can't go on spoiling your life any longer. I don't think two people could have been happier than we have been. V.[1]

No metaphor here, no sentimentality, no beating around the bush. She is desperately unhappy but, at the same time, straightforward in her desire to communicate. It's ironic that the momentum present in our rush to die can also contain the urgency to communicate. It's not that Woolf's suicide can be reduced to a lack of interpersonal communication. Seen from the perspective of a whole body-mind matrix, we can instead suggest that the parts that make up the sum of the body-mind/self were not communicating, not intimate, not grounded, felt, and made into words.

For someone pressed with visions and hearing voices, the key is using the frame of the body as an anchor to the present moment. Settling the mind not through using more narratives and thoughts but by turning to the body and breath is the key to the real feelings below the strategies of suicide. When we come right down to it, the core of what we feel is below the surface strategies of mind. In fact, the mind obsessed with death is not really that different from the compulsive mind most of us are working with every day. A mind spinning in its own solipsistic networks, cut off from the rhythm and feeling of body and breath, is self-identified with its pain and scars and perhaps even unwilling to part with them. We are easily attached to our misery by virtue of its being familiar. It's an easy way to define ourselves.

There is a parallel text to every story. Though someone is plagued with pain, the desire to end one's life is actually a counterpull against the identification with suffering. Suicide is the imagining of an end to suffering—an end that is certainly needed. Seeing more metaphorically, the desire for death as an end to suffering is a desire to make life more possible. What are we really hearing when we listen to fantasies of death? This is the energy—indeed, the paradox—I'd like to explore.

* * * * *

Yoga works in terms of complementary opposites. If you want to settle your inhalation, you spend time getting your exhalation very smooth; if you want to find extension in the hamstring muscles, you refine the contraction of the front of the thigh; if you want to find happiness, you serve others. Inside a forward bend is the seed of a backbend; in the midst of anxiety, we look for the calmness of the breath—it's always there.

Likewise, when we pay attention to the movement toward taking one's life, we also find the desire to live. This desire to live is expressed in the desire to communicate. The trick is dropping our preconceptions sufficiently to recognize this instinct, this movement *toward* intimacy. Even as the old tree withers and dies, we can find small emblems of growth. Illness, both mental and physical, often separates the afflicted from the world. Yoga reawakens one's connection with the whole body and mind and in so doing restores pathways of communication at an inner level that then begin to spread out into the interpersonal world as well. When we are safe in our own bodies, we have a ground from which to step out into the world.

Talking is a way of reaching something not clearly seen, verbally navigating through the fog of uncertainty. The problem with our Western perspective on suicide is that it's hard to listen when our very deliberate focus is on trying to stop someone from taking his own life, stop the urge toward death, protect ourselves from the legal repercussions of not calling the police. Since we all walk this same winding road toward death, someone else's desire to die brings up our own core ideas about death, dying, and what it means to live life fully.

Suicide in the Judeo-Christian perspective is rejected as sinful. In the early teachings of the Buddha, there are many stories of people like Channa, Vakkali, and Godhika, who took their own lives and were not condemned for it. If there is a cultural view that sees life as continuous in one way or another, especially if there is no god that determines whether someone is born again or not, we have permission to reframe our conceptualization of suicide as sinful. Who are we to judge?

Suicide is an internal drama that needs expression for it to be resolved. Suicide and self-harm must be understood as having meaning within interpersonal and intrapsychic relationships that the person is involved in. Wanting to die *means* something. What wants to die?

The problem with the "I"-making mechanism of the mind (*ahaṅkāra*) is that it creates stories (*asmitā*) that objectify itself. The "I" maker is constantly representing itself to itself, splitting the personality into a subject and object. This splits the *ahaṅkāra* into a storyteller that is telling itself a story by representing itself to itself. The core teachings of Yoga revolve around this case of mistaken identity. Any self-image is an objectification of the *ahaṅkāra* that serves to split the personality. If we understand the *ahaṅkāra* in this way, we can see that when one tells a story about oneself to oneself, one creates several selves. The ego can objectify itself.

The task for the yogi is to pay attention to life in ways that continually undercut our craving to have a fixed point of view. All sorts of things happen in our lives, tragedies and miracles together. We lose what we love and are continually separated from what we want. This is the way life goes. But this careful attention to the way our lives truly happen does not always go along with the therapeutic intention to "help life go on," "contract for safety," or "provide ego support." A focus on the absurd, the messy, the tragic, and the shameful parts of us is what's truly needed to open to our lives. With the help of a therapist, we can open to what we feel without fear. The key is being able to open to what we really feel, not just what we are allowed to feel either by our own internal judge or the unexamined assumptions in the medical stance of the clinician. Focusing on the body without searching for a way out can sometimes open up astonishing meaning within very old habits. We may even learn that the voice from the part of us that wants to die is exactly the same as the part of us that wants to come out into the world. The one who wants to die may really want to live after all. The "cry for help" is really a gesture to go through life with deep meaning and resolve. Wanting to die stands neither for life nor for death but for a deep experience of both of these opposites. To live is to allow for fixed views to die. To die is to be generous in our living.

In fantasies of suicide, the world becomes "outside" and separate from "me." The world shrinks to the small action of "me" and "my death." This is a selfish importance that can only be healed through returning back to a lived body, a network of relations, a life filled with meaning that comes through embodied experience, not through more storytelling. The selfishness of suicide is, however, a small seed of selfhood.

By processing the desire to die through staying close to what the patient feels in his or her body, we bring up insight into impermanence, showing us how what we feel is changing. What we desire in one moment becomes something entirely different in the next. The desire to jump gives way to a fantasy of wanting to find a husband, a better job, a more meaningful community. A seed must be closed tightly within itself in order to finally blossom. In this way the body of the therapist and the body of the patient enter despair together. The pain of the patient is fully felt by the therapist, and the patient is thus encouraged to face his or her overwhelming desire for the transcendent, the absolute, the eternal. Our deepest transformations occur when there is no hope, where nothing is left, not even the desire to live. Yet there is only *this* moment. A death in the future is not engagement with *this actual* experience *now*. It's a projection into the future.

What's disturbing about this is that the "I" maker (*ahaṅkāra*) can be overwhelmed by the selves it has created. Those selves are real, as real as any story we tell. But can we truly listen to these selves in a way that they can express themselves and begin moving toward wholeness again?

When we create space for free listening, we make room for free speech. We also make room for a wider spectrum of feelings. When we don't play the same records over and over, we reroot our openness of body and heart, allowing feelings and thoughts to move through awareness with less clinging. In the chains of words and ideas that come forth when we can hold the space of listening without judgment, the person in pain often has a surprising discovery, a spontaneous new arrival of insight that can only happen in the creative space of held silence. If we do not believe that the unconscious blocks that repress the expression of feeling can be supported by nonjudgmental listening, then we fall into the violent medical mentality that your symptoms are just functions of the brain. And if everything is a function of the brain, symptoms have no meaningful purpose. We need to rediscover our relation to the power of accompanied silence, of free listening, of self-expression. Again, the wish "to be dead" is a wish to attain peace and security at a time when one feels exactly the opposite. Every year, worldwide, an estimated three-quarters of a million people take their own life, making suicide and attempted suicide subjects we need to explore with much more creativity and interest.

Suicide is an attempt to resolve feelings of being overwhelmed by one's own image of oneself, or part of oneself. Suicide is an attack on one's own representation of one's body as an object. It's as if the death of the body can help one get rid of intolerable mental states and feelings. Suicide is a cry for help. Paying attention to this cry is practicing pain dharma, friendship dharma, and patience dharma.

If we value the subjective experience of the person, can we let go of our fixed personal, cultural, and professional ideas about death and listen to the truth of the inner turmoil of that individual?

Bearing witness requires that we put aside our fixed views. In this context bearing witness is experiencing the inner life of another, opening to our own feelings about what's showing up, eventually leading to compassionate action. The action we take, our moment of authenticity, requires courage, and we may have to bear the results of our courage and action. From the Yoga perspective, as soon as we speak of action, we're talking about ethics, because action always has a consequence both internally and externally.

If the primary motivation for taking action is *ahiṁsā*—not having the intention to cause harm to body, speech, or mind—how is suicide reconciled as an action?

To acknowledge one's intention is never simple. This is as true for the person feeling pain as it is for the one helping her. It requires willingness to take responsibility and recognize this ambivalence.

I feel traditional therapy is misguided on so many fronts, not the least of which is knowing how to work with the mind. A therapist should not simply identify or recognize patterns but move from knowing *about* something to actually allowing it to simply be.

Going back into the past often misses the functioning of the symptom in the present. The past is past. The past can only be experienced now. The past is what the mind is doing in present experience. A patient exploring suicide is exploring his or her pain in the present, and the past is encoded in the present. The hard work of the therapist is just to listen and explore what is present, not what is past. If it's not present, it's not here.

As a caricature, psychoanalysis ceases to be a study of identity and becomes instead an exploration of traumatic memories—it becomes, absurdly, an exercise in "proving" causal links between particular traumatic experiences and particular symptoms. This, of course, gives rise to the famous problem of the analyst's "suggesting" particular memories to the client.

Someone entertaining suicide is not only talking about future death. She is talking about present suffering. She is not describing historical trauma but rather current suffering. Suicide is not only a natural psychic reflex for surviving actual helplessness but is also an abstraction. We don't know what death will be like, only that something must be able to lift us out of this present and persistent pain. We need theories and abstractions about death, partly because the feelings that come up around suicide are so painful. Our theories and abstractions make the pain more bearable to us. The effect of embracing death and feeling what lies below our fantasies of our own termination brings about, at a critical moment, a radical transformation. The experience of looking deeply into death is a requisite for an engaged life. This implies that the crisis of suicide is a necessary phase in the life of any of us. Suicide itself may be too quick a transformation. The job of Yoga technique is to meditate on what is going on in the felt body in order to slow a hasty charge toward death and anchor us back in life.

Suicide is yelling out: "Life must change; Something must shift; I can't do this any longer. Having tried to change everything 'out there,' the only thing that can now change is inside me." And so suicide is a quick termination of what is so painful inside. The body, however, can be called in at this crucial junction. Attentiveness to the body dissolves this false dichotomy between inner and outer, me and not me. When we tune in to the breath, we tune in to life here and now. Life here and now is changing, and so there is no fixed self anywhere to be seen. This opens us up to change, freedom, and flexibility. Suicide is an attempt to move from one place to another through force. But force is exactly what got us into this mess to begin with. To force the body, the world, or ourselves into one frame is a kind of violence. Opening to change, through the body, unfixes us and paradoxically grounds us in the flowing conditions of our lives.

In the *Yoga Vasiṣṭha,* there is a wonderful moment during the dialogue between Vasiṣṭha and Rama concerning the way we cause suffering for ourselves where Vasiṣṭha declares: "The mind experiences what it itself has projected out of itself. By that it is bound."[2]

A young man who was contemplating suicide came to see me. His sister, who was studying Yoga at our center, recommended that he visit. He was estranged from his family and had nobody to turn to.

He showed up early for our first meeting, and his eyes never left mine. He sat forward in his chair and seemed eager to talk about what he was planning.

I asked him how he was going to find the pills he needed. He was shocked that I was prepared to talk about death, as he described it, "all the way."

"Yes," I said, "I am with you all the way."

"No," he demanded, "you can't be, because all the way is all the way and you won't be there."

"But I am here," I said.

"But that's not all the way."

"It is, though, it is all the way," I said, almost protesting.

"How is it all the way?"

"Well, I am here with you now. I can talk about this with you, plan it, listen to you. I understand. I have felt this pain."

"You can't feel what I feel."

"No, I can't. I can't ever feel what you feel. But I know pain, and I know that pain changes. I know that pain is deadly. I know you know that, too."

"Pain is not deadly, I am deadly."

"I don't understand."

"Pain is pain. Deadly is me. I am dead."

"If you are dead now, what have you got to lose?"

Suddenly, and out of nowhere, we both smiled. We had each other cornered. But we also had each other. In a way we were arguing about death. And the arguing made us both feel alive.

In a sense I was asking him: who does this mad voice inside you belong to? But of course there is no way to answer that question. However, posing the question allowed us to investigate. This person did not take his own life. Six years later he is still in pain, still stressed, but working through his pain by making art and living with a wonderful woman. He wants to be a father.

In this heated conversation, the person with whom I was speaking moved from wishing to control the outcome of his life to wishing to communicate with me. This is the real healing factor in any kind of helping work.

Psychiatrists and psychologists often "contract for safety" with suicidal patients; these patients avoid hospitalization based on their assurances that they will contact their clinicians if the inclination to commit suicide overwhelms them. Contracts for safety, or suicide prevention contracts, ask the patient to make a commitment, either verbally or in writing, to avoid self-destructive behavior and to keep the clinician informed of any such suicidal impulses.

Such contracts don't work. The real safety contract is in the quality of our ability to communicate and accept each other. Refusal to sign a no-suicide contract does not necessarily indicate that the patient is in imminent danger of suicide, just as agreement to a contract does not mean that the risk of suicide and self-destructive behavior is lessened. The mental state of a patient is not static. Patients may have inconsistent and complex motivations for agreeing to or refusing a contract.

Suicide moves from being *one* option to being *the* option when meaninglessness grows. Suicide is an attractive and logical solution when the pain and suffering that one is experiencing can't be met in a way that offers relief. Internal hatred must be transfigured into love through communication. This is *ahiṁsā* in action. Likewise the Buddha said: "Hatred is never quelled by hatred in this world. It is quelled by love. This is an eternal truth."[3]

Especially for the caregiver or friend, seated meditation with concentration on breathing is the primary way to remain centered in the midst of turbulence. Under some conditions we must accept suicide.

Skillfully, like the Buddha, we take advantage of each context to wake up. After Channa takes his own life, the Buddha says: "Without reproach was the knife used by the brother Channa."[4]

The Buddha is not condoning suicide. He is exonerating Channa. Can we do the same? Can we take each person's story to heart, one by one by one? Can we hear the pain of our friend who is dying to die? What can we offer? What good is it to blame or introduce anything other than loving action?

The practice of *ahiṁsā* is not to kill another living creature. But we do this every time we eat or pick our vegetables. Through a longer chain of causality, we do it every time we buy petroleum. One of the ways we take life is by not listening, by shutting down, by imposing our expectation on others. Someone who is in pain needs to be heard. Someone who wants to take her own life and is telling you about it desperately wants to connect, desperately desires intimacy. And you are there, in that moment, as best you can, to offer it. To offer yourself. Sometimes we think we know what a cry means, and sometimes we can't know. But we can put our bodies right there in the center of suffering and know it fully and mutually.

A therapist rooted in nonharming understands that when someone who wants to die is sitting face-to-face with you, that person is you. The first teachings around nonharm mean that we drop our expectations and favorite ways of doing things, we lay aside our viewpoint and professional obligation, and we serve someone exactly as he or she is. You can't preset the rules for this.

If someone is speaking to us as a therapist or friend or sibling, can we meet them *exactly* where they are? Can we continually check in with ourselves: what is going on now? If I am distracted, what is my most believed thought? Then we can return to our body and breath and then back to the person with whom we are working. We can't forget that the fundamental lesson of this yogic path is that difficult and even painful feelings are our opportunity to wake up to a more genuine way of living. This is as true for the person in pain as it is for the clinician or friend. We can always love more and more deeply.

Yogic ethics rely heavily on awareness practice, because if we can't return to this live moment, we are caught up in our theoretical understanding of the situation or in hope or fear. What is appropriate in one context may not be appropriate in another. Ethics are always a dialogue between our cultural background, our ability to open to present experience, and our individual ethical conscience.

It's amazing how our ethical conscience changes over time. Usually we can bring only a certain percentage of awareness to a situation, and then the unconscious ideals of the culture and our own past conditioning come in as a default position. One of the ways we can bring stable integrity and wisdom to our approach to someone in dire straits is to work with our fear of death.

The more we fear death, the more we accrue our basic narcissism. If we are trying to keep someone alive who wants to die, we are closing down the possible expression of some major knot now coming to the surface in that person's life (and by extension, in our own lives as well). A culture that hides, sanitizes, and represses death and dying is a culture afraid of its own mortality, thus setting up a world where heroic ambition, persona, and competitive self-interest are the most rewarded values.

This is imbalanced. The greatest attachment we all have to work through, Patañjali reminds us again and again, is *abiniveśa*, the fear of letting go of our clinging to the life of I, me, and mine.

Our attitude toward death is a central factor in the healing process because it influences the way we perceive life. With someone wanting to die, we don't know how to talk about death because we don't want to influence them one way or the other. But my experience is that time and time again, opening up the topic of death allows the person with whom we engaged to speak freely and openly without expectation.

Chögyam Trungpa says that when we go as far as we can in imagining and talking about death, some real sanity develops.[5]

It is much healthier to explore the psyche's ambivalent and twisted desires than it is to clean up the warehouse of the mind so it's all sanitized and perfect. How we act is in every way influenced by the all-embracing awareness and tenderness we can bring to the unconscious habit energies and turbulence of mind and body.

Suicide is not just death's call. It's a wake-up call.

This is an entirely practical approach. What's going on right now? What is this person saying? How am I listening? These questions are a matter of value: do we value our ideas that one should live and be healthy or do we most value what is occurring in this very moment? When we give up our ideas about value, ironically, things become meaningful. In this way, there is no zone of comfort, but there is the marvelous flux of intimacy out of which healing is possible.

When we begin to take these teachings seriously—when we look directly at the truth of impermanence, the movement of the *gunas* (qualities of nature), the stability of awareness, the emptiness of self-image—we learn that the most practical tool of awakening is giving up the task of looking for certainty. When we place burdens and cultural expectations on others, especially those in need, we are setting a bar that nobody can or should ever live up to. Expectations are the roots of violence. When we give up our desire to be helpful, to help others to live, even to want life to go on for a young person in need, we can drop right into the unfolding flow of life as it really is.

Life as it really is contains both the transcendent and the imminent, both phases of joy and phases of discontent. The moral tragedy of the satifaction-dissatisfaction cycle is that it sometimes makes life feel impossible. When I recently learned that author David Foster Wallace hung himself in the suburban garage in which he wrote, I felt a kind of relief. A tension had been building in me while I explored his work. He struggled so much with a superior intellect and a creative and solipsistic mental life. For reasons we can never know, it became too much for him. He tried. He sought help. He changed his writing styles over and over again—he included lengthy footnotes to deal with his tangential thought process and endless elaborations. Who am I to judge his actions? I miss him here in the community of writers I admire. I also relate to his struggle.

The base or substance of life, like the substratum we call silence, is not a blank nothingness but an interwoven fullness, a brightness, a roaring murmur of activity. In the absence of so much chattering and knowing about this and that, there is no collapsing vacuum. Instead, we begin to see that solutions don't come from isolating ourselves from the circumstances of our lives and our bodies. Life comes to feel precious not in an individualized way but as some inexplicable part of a larger whole. When we lose sight of how each moment of our lives is a resonant connection with all of life, regardless of whether it is pleasant or painful, we will continually yearn for something else, even finality. The dharma, friendship, and trusting in the body and breath help free us from being overidentified with our symptoms.

There is no security against death. We can imagine the moment of death as a rebirth into new form. Death is both a discontinuity and continuity. The one we love and know discontinues, yet the fluids and flesh return to earth again and begin a new life. At death we do not slip into nothingness—we slip into existence. The waves become the water once again.

For the person who wants to die, the horror is that his demons *refuse* to die. Madness would be an easier escape, but he is not wired to go mad, he is wired to bear his pain. The sheer weight of these inner demands needs attention, but sometimes the personality is not strong enough or not skilled in knowing how to listen. A third ear is needed: a companion, a mother. The world is the only reality of which we can be sure, but if the world is unbearable, if he can't bear the pain alone, who are we to judge? Having made the decision to die, he lives his truth by refusing to live in the world. From the perspective of Yoga, his death is impossible.

In describing his own suicidal fantasies, poet Jim Harrison writes with rare eloquence and poignancy:

Beauty takes my courage away this cold autumn evening. My year-old daughter's red robe hangs from the doorknob shouting *Stop*.[6]

Halifax, Nova Scotia, and Cape Cod, Massachusetts, 2008

AFTERWORD

WHENEVER WE OPEN our mouths, an old Japanese saying goes, we always get mud on our face. Of course this is true in the realm of language, in the exposition of our ideas in this stumbling realm of words and speech. The nucleus of spiritual practice is twofold: internal quietude and expression. Like inhaling and exhaling, these two activities are complementary opposites. Love, compassion, wisdom—these are simply the connecting forces that occur when both stillness and expression are present. Stillness is not just sitting under a tree with eyes fixed on the horizon of the grass and shrubs and mind but includes the thoughtfulness in our speech and the quietness of a mind committed in activity.

To see how our experience is unconstructed through stillness is a profound experience because we can learn how much of our lives happens below auspices of the discriminating mind. Touching this receptive place of *samādhi* can give us a deep faith in quiet, long-term practice because we begin to see just how much trouble we make for ourselves! The world is immense. Linguistic structures constantly force distinctions in our lives until we realize that the old sages like Patañjali were absolutely right. We need to begin in the body and corporeal world so that the mind can quiet and learn to see things in clear and precise dimensions. The Yoga postures are an art form when striving is absent, and the breathing techniques of *Śiva Saṁhitā* and other great texts are like the textbooks that refine our attention and the nervous system. Our cities and our friends are the canvas on which we express our practice—it is through community and self-expression that service becomes creative and vital in our everyday lives.

Over the five years of teachings that occurred during the talks collected in this small anthology, I rarely prepared notes or thoughts beforehand. Yoga teacher Richard Freeman once told me that when he gives a talk he "simply speaks about whatever is happening in the room." I always prepare a poem or a *sūtra* and use that as a basis for the talks. When the room is full, like a bustling Tuesday evening at Centre of Gravity in Toronto, I try to match whatever I am working with in my own practice with what I feel is happening in the room at that moment.

I like teaching mothers and fathers, artists and musicians, activists and those who are thinking through the way their lives can be transformed into skillful paths of service.

Sometimes doubt shows up in our practice as a complementary twin to the faith that dedicated practice requires. Studying old texts and practicing what's described by living teachers helps us see through the doubts so that indecision and waffling don't get the better of our practice time. The doubt that is most healthy in our practice is not doubting the teaching as much as doubting the person who is listening and breathing and reading these very sentences. This practice aims at that person. Who is breathing? Who is reading?

I am rereading these essays over a week of teaching in Montreal, Brooklyn, and the mountains of British Columbia. Sometimes I want to go back and change so many things that are now on paper, that now have a small ledge in history. These teachings may be universal, but they also need to adapt to the conditions of our lives. I love these practices. Sometimes during retreats, I find myself overwhelmed by the joy of walking meditation, interviews, and even setting the hall up with rows and rows of zafus and zabutons, mats and blocks and straps.

May your life go well.

Montreal, 2009

ACKNOWLEDGMENTS

AFTER INTERVIEWING ME for an article entitled "Anarchy Yoga" in the now defunct *Ascent* magazine, Christopher McCann and I spoke of editing a large box of transcribed dharma talks in order to capture the philosophical, cultural, and political dimensions of Yoga practice. Chris went to work and did an excellent job arranging them in an order that made sense. Again, Emily Bower and the team at Shambhala have brought another book (number four) into the world in the same number of years. Sarah Selecky took the final manuscript and reworked the grainy sections in ways that I couldn't see for myself. Sarah's writing and editing guidance have been profound. Elaine Jackson edited the final manuscript.

Thank you to my teachers, Norman Feldman and Enkyo Roshi.

Anthony Wilson has provided invaluable heartfelt guidance to me for many years.

I am continually surprised by how much energy I have for teaching, study, and practice, and much of this comes from my love of the dharma but most especially from the support and process of the wonderful communities both in Toronto and abroad that I've come to know over the years. Although these talks appear in this book as formal and finalized comments, they are the product of endless conversations, debate, and discussion. You, the reader, complete each one of these talks when you express what you've learned through action.

My son has unknowingly brought these teachings home to me in an everyday way, and to him this book is dedicated. My uncle Ian Eckler was my first Yoga teacher, and he too has influenced every page of this collection.

NOTES

1. This Is It

1. Quoted by Robert Aitken in "Taking Responsibility," an address to the Buddhist Peace Fellowship Membership Gathering, June 23, 2006, http://www.thezensite.com/ZenTeachings/Miscellaneous/Aitken_on_Responsibility.pdf.

3. The Realization of Intimacy

1. Tīrthāvalī, quoted by Christian Lee Novetzke in "A Family Affair: Krishna Comes to Paṇḍharpūr and Makes Himself at Home," quoted in Guy L. Beck, ed., *Alternative Krishnas: Regional and Vernacular Variations on a Hindu Deity* (Albany: State University of New York Press, 2005), 123.
2. William James, *The Principles of Psychology* (New York: Holt, 1890), quoted in John Welwood, *Toward a Psychology of Awakening* (Boston: Shambhala Publications, 2000), 44.
3. Ibid., 45.
4. Virginia Woolf, "A Sketch of the Past," in *Moments of Being* (Ann Arbor: University of Michigan Press/Harcourt Brace Jovanovich, 1976), 101.

4. The Breath Cycle

1. Zoketsu Norman Fischer, introduction to *Beyond Thinking: Meditation Guide by Zen Master Dogen,* trans. by Kazuaki Tanahashi (Boston: Shambhala Publications, 2004), xxvii.

5. The Object of Meditation

1. Chip Hartranft, trans., *The Yoga-Sūtra of Patañjali* (Boston: Shambhala Publications, 2003), 3.1–10.
2. *Yoga-Sūtra*, 3.1–7, my translation. See also Hartranft, 3.1–7.
3. Ibid., 2.45–46.
4. Ibid., 2.46–47.
5. Leonard Cohen, "S.O.S. 1995," in *Book of Longing* (Toronto: McClelland and Stewart, 2006), 8.

8. Not Closing Our Eyes

1. Sigmund Freud, *Studies on Hysteria* (1893), in *Selected Papers on Hysteria and Other Psychoneuroses,* trans. by A. A. Brill (New York: Journal of Nervous and Mental Disease Publishing Company, 1912); www.bartleby.com/280.
2. Ibid.
3. Ibid.

9. Ontario Snow Lineage

1. Hartranft, *Yoga-Sūtra*, 1.3.

10. Liberation

1. *Yoga-Sūtra,* 2.51–52, my translation.
2. For more information on these authors in relation to Buddhist thought, see David Loy, *Lack and Transcendence* (Amherst, Mass.: Humanity Books, 1996).
3. *Yoga-Sūtra,* 1.4, my translation.

11. The Life of a Tulip

1. Abu Taleb, "Travels," 1:218–20, quoted in Stephen Hay, ed., *Sources of Indian Tradition* (New York: Columbia University Press, 1988), 13.

2. *Sutta Nipata* (Group of Discourses), trans. Nanavira Thera, in *The Group of Discourses,* 2d ed. K. R. Norman, ed. (Oxford, U.K.: Pali Text Society, 2001), 651–53.

3. *Dhammapada,* p. 80, trans. by Stephen Batchelor, personal communication, Toronto, 2010, unpublished, used with permission.

4. Bhikku Bodhi, trans., *Connected Discourses of the Buddha: A New Translation of the Samyutta Nikaya,* S. IV 229–31, (Boston: Wisdom Publications, 2000).

5. *Majjhima Nikaya* 131, Bhaddekaratta Sutta: An Auspicious Day, translated from the Pali by Thanissaro Bhikkhu, www.accesstoinsight.org/tipitaka/mn/mn.131.than.html, accessed November 2010.

6. Śāntideva, *The Bodhicaryāvatāra,* VIII.26, 28, trans. Kate Crosby and Andrew Skilton (Oxford: Oxford University Press, 1996), 90.

7. Dalai Lama, "Dalai Lama says climate change needs global action," www.tibet.net/en/index.php. Article is no longer accessible.

8. For a contemporary discussion on the axial-age civilizations, see Shmuel N. Eisenstadt, ed., *The Origins and Diversity of Axial-Age Civilizations* (Albany: State University of New York Press, 1986).

9. Chang Tsai (Zhang Zai), "The Western Inscription," in Wing-tsit Chan, trans., *A Source Book in Chinese Philosophy* (Princeton: Princeton University Press, 1963), 497.

10. http://hdr.undp.org/en/humandev/forum/1999/agenda/, accessed 2004.

12. Diversity

1. Paul Hawken, *Blessed Unrest* (New York: Viking, 2007), 71.

2. *Puruṣa Sūkta,* my own translation, Ṛg Veda x:190, 13-14.

3. Robert Ernest Hume, trans., *The Thirteen Principal Upaniṣads* (Oxford: Oxford University Press, 1931); *Bṛadāraṇyaka*

Upaniṣad III:9.28, quoted in Christopher Key Chapple, *Nonviolence to Animals, Earth, and Self in Asian Traditions* (Albany: State University of New York Press, 1999), 51.

4. Hawken, *Blessed Unrest,* 71–72.

5. *Yoga-Sūtra,* 2.48, my own translation.

13. WAVES AND WATER: FORM AND FREEDOM

1. Hikai no Go, *Yamato Monogatari* (Tale of Yamato), quoted in Kenneth Yasuda, *The Japanese Haiku* (Japan: Charles E. Tuttle, 1957), 127.

2. "Dokugo Shingyo: Acid Comments on the Heart Sutra by Hakuin," http://members.optushome.com.au/davidquinn000/ Hakuin%20folder/Hakuin09.html. Accessed October 2010.

3. Sigmund Freud, "Beyond the Pleasure Principle," in *On Metapsychology* (Middlesex, England: Penguin, 1991), 278.

4. "The True Path," in *Zen Flesh, Zen Bones,* ed. Paul Reps and Nyogen Sensei (Boston: Tuttle Publishing, 1998), 71.

5. Gerry Wick, *The Book of Equanimity* (Somerville, Mass.: Wisdom Publications, 2005), 300.

6. When we try to consolidate this flow of life into a persona or a belief system, we become caught in the virtual reality of suffering, of conditioned knowledge. We forget, as it's said in the *Chāndogya Upaniṣad* (7.25.2), that "The self, indeed, is the whole world." Or in the *Muṇḍaka Upaniṣad* (2.2.11), "The true reality (Brahman), indeed, is this whole world, this widest extent."

7. Swami Venkatesanda, *The Supreme Yoga: A New Transaltion of the Yoga Vasista,* vol. 1 (Uttar Pradesh, India: The Divine Life Society, 1976), 215.

8. Meiko Matsudaira, "Passion unspoken/ . . . ," in Leza Lowitz, Miyuki Aoyama, and Akemi Tomioka, eds., *A Long Rainy Season: Haiku and Tanka: Contemporary Japanese Women's Poetry,* vol. 1 (Berkeley, Calif.: Stone Bridge Press, 1994).

14. Encouragement on Retreat

1. *Yoga-Sūtra* 10.58, 1, 3–9, 12. This is my own reworking of the excellent translation by Wendy Doniger in *The Rig Veda* (London: Penguin Classics, 1981).
2. Traditional Vedic chant taught to me one-on-one by Pandit Guar, Fern Street Hindu temple, Toronto, January 2005.

15. End of Retreat

1. Victor H. Mair, trans., *Tao Te Ching* (New York: Bantam Books, 1990), 60; also see chap. 67.
2. My own translation of the Bhagavad-Gītā, 18.11-12, based on Juan Mascaro, trans., *The Bhagavad-Gītā* (London: Penguin Books, 1962).
3. "Bodaisatta Shishoho" (The Four Integrative Methods of Bodhisattvas), in *Shobogenzo: Zen Essays by Dōgen,* trans. Thomas Cleary (Honolulu: University of Hawaii Press, 1986), 119. Also see Kosen Nishiyama and John Stevens, *A Complete English Translation of Dōgen Zenjui's Shōbōgenzo,* vol. 3, 117 (no. 11) (San Francisco: Japan Publications Trading Company, 1975).
4. Hartranft, *Yoga-Sūtra,* 3.2.
5. *The Heart Sutra,* trans. Red Pine (Berkeley, Calif.: Shoemaker & Hoard, 2005).
6. Stephen Batchelor, *Alone with Others* (New York: Grove Press, 1983), 105.

16. The Nonduality of Inner and Outer Practice

1. *Yoga-Sūtra,* 2.29. My translation.
2. "Talk when you talk/ . . . ," from "Gospel Noble Truths" in Allen Ginsberg, *Collected Poems, 1947–1980,* (San Francisco: HarperCollins, 1975).

17. Money and the Turnings of Mind

1. Zen handout (Rochester, N.Y.: Rochester Zen Center, 1988).
2. Giovanni Pico della Mirandola, *Oration on the Dignity of Man,* trans. Aloysius Robert Caponigri (Chicago: Regnery Gateway, 1956; reprint Washington: Regnery Publishing, 1996).
3. David Loy, personal communcation, 2007.

18. Activism with Both Feet on the Ground

1. Hartranft, *Yoga-Sūtra,* 1.30–35.
2. Charles Darwin, quoted in Adam Phillips, *Darwin's Worms* (New York: Basic Books, 2000), 58.
3. Paul Hawken, "Taking the Natural Step," *In Context* (Context Institute, 1995), www.context.org/ICLIB/IC41/Hawken2.htm.
4. Mihaly Csikszentmihalyi, *The Evolving Self* (New York: Harper Collins, 1993), 18.
5. Ibid., 19.
6. Śaṅkara, *Vivekacūḍāmaṇi,* trans. Madhavananda (Calcutta: Advaita Ashrama, 1974), 194.

19. The Lungs of the Earth

1. Karen Armstrong, *Buddha* (Toronto: Penguin, 2004).
2. Rainforest Action Network, www.ran.org/info_center/about_rainforests.html.
3. Edward Hoagland, "Endgame," *Harpers* (June 2007): 42.
4. *Yoga-Sūtra,* 1.43, my translation.
5. Ibid, 4.23–24.
6. Śaṅkarācārya, in Juliana Horatia Gatty Ewing, ed., *The Ve-danta-Sutras with the Commentary by Sankaracarya, Sacred Books of the East* (1883), vol. 1 (Boston: Adamant Media Corporation, 2000).

7. Buddhagosa, *Sāratthapakāsinī* 2.99, quoted in David Kalupahana, *Causality: The Central Philosophy of Buddhism* (Honolulu: University of Hawaii Press, 1975), 83.

8. Hartranft, 2.9.

9. Arne Naess, "Identification as a Source of Deep Ecological Attitudes," in Michael Tobias, ed., *Deep Ecology,* 2d revised ed. (San Francisco: Pfeiffer, 1985).

10. John Seed, "The Ecological Self," *The Trumpeter* 22, no. 2 (2006). Available at http://trumpeter.athabascau.ca/index.php/ trumpet/article/view/909/1341. Accessed November 2010. See also Anthony Weston, "Non-Anthropocentrism in a Thoroughly Anthropocentrized World," *The Trumpeter* 8, no. 3 (1991). Available at http://trumpeter.athabascau.ca/index.php/ trumpet/article/view/459/761. Accessed November 2010.

11. William James, "The Empirical Self," in *Principles of Psychology,* quoted by Arne Naess in "Identification as a Source of Deep Ecological Attitudes" in *Deep Ecology,* ed. Michael Tobias (Boston: Pfeiffer, 1985), 259.

20. Suicide

1. Phyllis Rose, *Woman of Letters: A Life of Virginia Woolf* (Oxford: Routledge, 1986), 243.

2. Venkatesananda and Christopher Chapple, trans., *The Concise Yoga Vāsiṣṭha* (New York: SUNY Press, 1985), chap. 4.

3. Acharya Buddharakkhita, trans., "Yamakavagga: Pairs," www .accesstoinsight.org/tipitaka/kn/dhp/dhp.01.budd.html.

4. F. L. Woodward, *Kindred Sayings,* vol. 4 (Somerville, Mass.: Wisdom Publications, 1980), 33.

5. Chögyam Trungpa, *The Heart of the Buddha* (Boston: Shambhala Publications, 1991), 178.

6. Jim Harrison, *Letters to Yesenin* (Port Townsend, Wash.: Copper Canyon Press, 1973), 6.

CREDITS

INDEX